Environmental Health Criteria 112

TRI-*n*-BUTYL PHOSPHATE

Published under the joint sponsorship of the United Nations Environment Programme, the International Labour Organisation, and the World Health Organization

First draft prepared by Dr A. Nakamura, National Institute for Hygienic Sciences, Japan

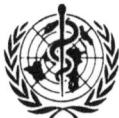

World Health Organization
Geneva, 1991

The **International Programme on Chemical Safety (IPCS)** is a joint venture of the United Nations Environment Programme, the International Labour Organisation, and the World Health Organization. The main objective of the IPCS is to carry out and disseminate evaluations of the effects of chemicals on human health and the quality of the environment. Supporting activities include the development of epidemiological, experimental laboratory, and risk-assessment methods that could produce internationally comparable results, and the development of manpower in the field of toxicology. Other activities carried out by the IPCS include the development of know-how for coping with chemical accidents, coordination of laboratory testing and epidemiological studies, and promotion of research on the mechanisms of the biological action of chemicals.

WHO Library Cataloguing in Publication Data

Tri-*n*-butyl phosphate.

(Environmental health criteria ; 112)

1. Phosphoric acid esters - adverse effects
2. Phosphoric acid esters - toxicity
I. Series

ISBN 92 4 157112 8   (NLM Classification: QV 627)
ISSN 0250-863X

©World Health Organization 1991

Printed in Finland
DHSS — Vammala — 5000

CONTENTS

ENVIRONMENTAL HEALTH CRITERIA FOR TRI-*n*-BUTYL PHOSPHATE

WHO TASK GROUP ON ENVIRONMENTAL HEALTH CRITERIA FOR TRI-*n*-BUTYL PHOSPHATE

Members

Dr S. Dobson, Institute of Terrestrial Ecology, Monks Wood Experimental Station, Abbots Ripton, Huntingdon, Cambridgeshire, England (*Chairman*)

Dr S. Fairhurst, Medical Division, Health and Safety Executive, Bootle, Merseyside, England *(Joint Rapporteur)*

Ms N. Kanoh, Division of Information on Chemical Safety, National Institute of Hygienic Sciences, Setagaya-ku, Tokyo, Japan

Dr A. Nakamura, Division of Medical Devices, National Institute of Hygienic Sciences, Setagaya-ku, Tokyo, Japan

Dr M. Tasheva, Department of Toxicology, Institute of Hygiene and Occupational Health, Sofia, Bulgaria

Dr B. Veronesi, Neurotoxicology Division, US Environmental Protection Agency, Research Triangle Park, North Carolina, USA

Mr W.D. Wagner, Division of Standards Development and Technology Transfer, National Institute for Occupational Safety and Health, Cincinnati, Ohio, USA

Dr R. Wallentowicz, Exposure Assessment Application Branch, US Environmental Protection Agency, Washington, DC, USA (*Joint Rapporteur*)

Dr Shen-Zhi Zhang, Beijing Municipal Centre for Hygiene and Epidemic Control, Beijing, China

Observers

Dr M. Beth, Berufsgenossenschaft der Chemischen Industrie (BG Chemie), Heidelberg, Federal Republic of Germany

Dr R. Kleinstück, Bayer AG, Leverkusen, Federal Republic of Germany

Secretariat

Dr M. Gilbert, International Programme on Chemical Safety, Division of Environmental Health, World Health Organization, Switzerland (*Secretary*)

NOTE TO READERS OF THE CRITERIA DOCUMENTS

Every effort has been made to present information in the criteria documents as accurately as possible without unduly delaying their publication. In the interest of all users of the environmental health criteria documents, readers are kindly requested to communicate any errors that may have occurred to the Manager of the International Programme on Chemical Safety, World Health Organization, Geneva, Switzerland, in order that they may be included in corrigenda, which will appear in subsequent volumes.

* * *

A detailed data profile and a legal file can be obtained from the International Register of Potentially Toxic Chemicals, Palais des Nations, 1211 Geneva 10, Switzerland (Telephone No. 7988400 or 7985850).

ENVIRONMENTAL HEALTH CRITERIA FOR TRI-*n*-BUTYL PHOSPHATE

A WHO Task Group meeting on Environmental Health Criteria for Tri-*n*-butyl Phosphate was held at the British Industrial Biological Research Association (BIBRA), Carshalton, United Kingdom, from 9 to 13 October 1989. Dr S.D. Gangolli, Director, BIBRA, welcomed the participants on behalf of the host institution and Dr M. Gilbert opened the meeting on behalf of the three cooperating organizations of the IPCS (ILO, UNEP, WHO). The Task Group reviewed and revised the draft criteria document and made an evaluation of the risks for human health and the environment from exposure to tri-*n*-butyl phosphate.

The first draft of this document was prepared by Dr A. Nakamura, National Institute for Hygienic Sciences, Japan. Dr M. Gilbert and Dr P.G. Jenkins, both members of the IPCS Central Unit, were responsible for the overall scientific content and editing, respectively.

ABBREVIATIONS

BCF	bioconcentration factor
BUN	blood urea nitrogen
EC	effective concentration
FPD	flame photometric detector
GC	gas chromatography
GPC	gel permeation chromatography
HPLC	high performance liquid chromatography
LC	lethal concentration
LD	lethal dose
MS	mass spectrometry
NADPH	reduced nicotinamide adenine dinucleotide phosphate
NPD	nitrogen-phosphorus sensitive detector
OPIDN	organophosphate-induced delayed neuropathy
TAP	trialkyl/aryl phosphate
TBP	tri-n-butyl phosphate
TCP	tricresyl phosphate
TLC	thin-layer chromatography
TPP	triphenyl phosphate

1. SUMMARY

1.1 Identity, physical and chemical properties, analytical methods

Tri-*n*-butyl phosphate (TBP) is a non-flammable, non-explosive, colourless, odourless liquid. However, it is thermally unstable and begins to decompose at temperatures below its boiling point. By analogy with the known chemical properties of trimethyl phosphate, TBP is thought to hydrolyse readily in either acidic, neutral, or alkaline solutions. It behaves as a weak alkylating agent. The partition coefficient between octanol and water (log P_{ow}) is 3.99-4.01.

The analytical method of choice is gas-liquid chromatography with a nitrogen-phosphorus sensitive or flame photometric detector. The detection limit in water is about 50 ng/litre. Contamination of analytical reagents with TBP has been frequently reported; therefore, care must be taken in order to obtain reliable data in trace analysis of TBP.

1.2 Sources of human and environmental exposure

TBP is manufactured by the reaction of *n*-butanol with phosphorus oxychloride. It is used as a solvent for cellulose esters, lacquers, and natural gums, as a primary plasticizer in the manufacture of plastics and vinyl resins, as a metal extractant, as a base stock in the formulation of fire-resistant aircraft hydraulic fluids, and as an antifoaming agent. During the past few years, the utilization of TBP as an extractant in the dissolution process in conventional nuclear fuel reprocessing has increased considerably.

Exposure of the general population through normal use can be regarded as minimal.

1.3 Environmental transport, distribution, and transformation

When used as an extraction reagent, solvent, or antifoaming agent, TBP is continuously lost to the air and aquatic environment. The biodegradation of TBP is moderate or slow depending on the ratio of TBP to active biomass. It involves stepwise enzymatic hydrolysis to orthophosphate and *n*-butanol, which undergoes further degradation. The concentration of TBP in water is not decreased by standard techniques for drinking-water treatment.

Bioconcentration factors (BCF) measured for two species of fish (killifish and goldfish) range from 6 to 49. The depuration half-life was 1.25 h.

1.4 Environmental levels and human exposure

TBP has been found frequently in air, water, sediment, and aquatic organisms, but levels in environment samples are low. Higher concentrations of TBP have been detected in air, water, and fish samples collected near paper manufacturing plants in Japan: 13.4 ng/m^3 in air; 25 200 ng per litre in river water; 111 ng/g in fish organs. Total diet-studies in the United Kingdom and the USA indicate average daily TBP intakes of approximately 0.02-0.08 μg per kg body weight per day.

1.5 Effects on organisms in the environment

The inhibitory concentrations (EC_0, EC_{50}, EC_{100}) of TBP for the multiplication of unicellular algae, protozoa, and bacteria have been estimated to lie within the range of 3.2-100 mg/litre. The acute toxicity fish (LC_{50}) ranges from 4.2 to 11.8 mg/litre. TBP increases the drying rate of plant leaves, which results in rapid and complete inhibition of leaf respiration.

1.6 Kinetics and metabolism

In experimental animals, oral or intraperitoneally injected TBP is readily transformed by the liver, and presumably by the kidney, to yield hydroxylated products as butyl moieties. TBP is excreted mainly as dibutyl hydrogen phosphate, butyl dihydrogen phosphate, and butyl bis-(3-hydroxybutyl) phosphate. Alkyl moieties hydroxylated as alkyl chains are removed and excreted partly as *N*-acetylalkyl cysteine and partly as carbon dioxide.

1.7 Effects on experimental animals and *in vitro* test systems

Oral LD_{50} values for TBP in mice and rats have been reported to range from about 1 to 3 g/kg, indicating relatively low acute toxicity.

In subchronic toxicity studies with TBP, dose-dependent depression of body weight gain and increases in liver, kidney, and testis weights were reported. The results of the subchronic studies indicate that the kidney may be a target organ of TBP.

Primary skin irritation caused by TBP in albino rabbits may be as serious as that caused by morpholine.

TBP is reported to be slightly teratogenic at high dose levels. The mutagenicity of TBP has been inadequately investigated. Negative results have been reported in bacterial tests and in a recessive lethal mutation test with *Drosophila melanogaster*.

There are no adequate data to assess the carcinogenicity of TBP, and the effects on reproduction have not been investigated.

The ability of TBP to produce delayed neuropathy has been inadequately investigated. Effects seen following oral administration of a high dose (0.42 ml/kg per day for 14 days) suggested delayed neuropathy, but no axonal degeneration was seen and no definite conclusions could be drawn. This same high dose (0.42 ml/kg per day for 14 days) caused a significant reduction in conduction velocity of the caudal nerve and morphological alteration of unmyelinated fibres in rats. These results indicate that TBP has a neurotoxic effect on the peripheral nerve.

1.8 Effects on humans

In an *in vitro* study, TBP has been reported to have a slight inhibitory effect on human plasma cholinesterase.

There are no case reports of delayed neurotoxicity, as has been observed in cases of tri-*o*-cresyl phosphate poisoning.

2. IDENTITY, PHYSICAL AND CHEMICAL PROPERTIES, ANALYTICAL METHODS

2.1 Identity

Chemical Structure:

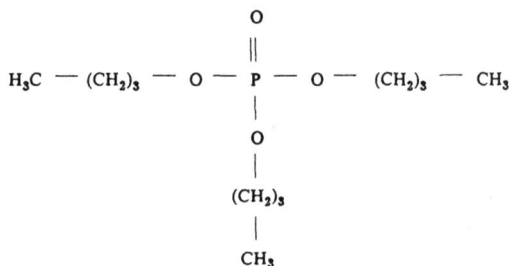

$$H_3C - (CH_2)_3 - O - \overset{\displaystyle O}{\underset{\displaystyle \underset{\displaystyle \underset{\displaystyle CH_3}{(CH_2)_3}}{O}}{\overset{\displaystyle \|}{P}}} - O - (CH_2)_3 - CH_3$$

Molecular formula: $C_{12}H_{27}O_4P$

Relative molecular mass: 266.3

CAS chemical name: Phosphoric acid, tributyl ester

CAS registry number: 126-73-8

RTECS registry number: TC7700000

Synonyms: TBP; tri-*n*-butyl phosphate; phosphoric acid, tri-*n*-butyl ester

Trade name: Phosflex 4®; Skydrol LD-4®; Celluphos 4®; Disphamol 1 TBP®

Manufacturers and suppliers (Modern Plastics Encyclopedia, 1975; Parker, 1980; Laham et al., 1984):
    Albright & Wilson Ltd.;
    A & K Petroleum Ind. Ltd. (Laham et al., 1984);
    Ashland Chemical Co.; Bayer AG;
    Commercial Solvent Corp.; East Coast Chemicals Co.;
    FMC Corporation; McKesson Chemical Co.;

Mobay Chemical Co.; Mobil Chemical Co.;
Monsanto Chemical Co.; Rhone-Poulenc Co.;
Protex (SA) Stauffer Chemical Co.; Tenneco
Organics Daihachi Chemical Ind. Co.; Nippon
Chemical Ind. Co. Ltd.

2.2 Physical and chemical properties

The physical properties of tri-*n*-butyl phosphate
(TBP) are listed in Table 1.

Table 1. Physical properties of tri-*n*-butyl phosphate

Physical state	colourless, odourless liquid
Melting point (°C)	-80[a]
Boiling point (°C)	289 (with decomp.)[b,d]; 177-178 (3.6 kPa)[b,d]; 150 (1.33 kPa)[b]
Flash point (°C)	193[b]; 166[a]; 146[d]
Relative density	0.973-0.983 (25 °C)[b]; 0.978 (20 °C)[a]
Refractive index	1.4226 (25 °C)[b]; 1.4215 (25 °C)[d]
Viscosity (cSt)	3.5-12.2[b]; 3.7[a]
Surface tension	29 dynes/cm (20 °C)
Vapour pressure	66.7 kPa (200 °C)[a]; 973 Pa (150 °C)[a] 133 Pa (100 °C)[c]; 9 Pa (25 °C)
Solubility in organic solvents	miscible with organic solvents
Solubility in water (mg/litre)	1012 (4 °C)[e]; 0.422 (25 °C)[e]; 2.85 x 10^{-4} (50 °C)[e]
Octanol-water partition coefficient (log P$_{ow}$)	4.00[f]; 3.99[g]; 4.01[h]

[a] Laham et al. (1984)
[b] Modern Plastics Encyclopedia (1975)
[c] Parker (1980)
[d] Windholz (1983)
[e] Higgins et al. (1959)
[f] Saeger et al. (1979)
[g] Sasaki et al. (1981)
[h] Kenmotsu et al. (1980b)

TBP is non-flammable and non-explosive. However, it
is thermally unstable and begins to decompose at temperatures below its boiling point (Paciorex et al., 1978;
Bruneau et al., 1981). The weak bond of the molecule is
the C-O bond, and its primary splitting leads to butene
and phosphoric acid (Bruneau et al., 1981). With an
excess of oxygen, complete combustion to carbon dioxide
and water occurs at about 700 °C (Bruneau et al., 1981).

Despite a lack of data, TBP is thought to hydrolyse readily in either acidic, neutral, or alkaline solution, based on the known chemical properties of trimethyl phosphate (Barnard et al., 1961).

2.3 Conversion factor

Tributyl phosphate   1 ppm = 10.89 mg/m^3

2.4 Analytical methods

Analytical methods for determining TBP in air, water, sediment, fish, and biological tissues are summarized in Table 2. The methods of choice are gas chromatography (GC) equipped with a nitrogen-phosphorus sensitive detector (GC/NPD) or flame photometric detector (GC/FPD), and gas chromatography plus mass spectrometry (GC/MS). The detection limit in water by GC/NPD or GC/FPD is approximately 50 ng/litre. TBP and other trialkyl/aryl phosphates (TAPs), e.g., triphenyl phosphate (TPP), trioctyl phosphate, and tricresyl phosphate (TCP), can be simultaneously determined by GC. Thin-layer chromatography (TLC) is sometimes used for determining TBP but is not widely applicable.

2.4.1 Extraction and concentration

TBP is easily extracted from aqueous solution with methylene chloride or benzene (Kenmotsu et al., 1980a; Kurosaki et al., 1983; Ishikawa et al., 1985). Low levels of TBP in water are successfully concentrated on Amberlite XAD-2 resin (Lebel et al., 1979, 1981), XAD-4 resin (Hutchins et al., 1983), or a mixed resin of XAD-4 and XAD-8 (Rossum & Webb, 1978). The purge-trap method with charcoal filter for ng/litre levels of TBP was reported by Grob & Grob (1974), but the percentage recovery was not calculated.

TBP may be extracted from sediment with polar solvents such as acetonitrile (Kenmotsu et al., 1980a) or acetone (Ishikawa et al., 1985).

Acetonitrile and methylene chloride (Kenmotsu et al., 1980a) or acetone-hexane (Lebel & Williams, 1983; EAJ, 1984) have been used for extracting TBP from fish or

Table 2. Methods for the determination of TBP

Sample type	Sampling method; extraction/clean-up	Analytical method[a]	Limit of detection	Comment	Reference
Environmental air	trap with glycerol-Florisil column, elute with methanol, add water, and extract with hexane	GC/FPD	1 ng/m^3	simultaneous method for trialkyl/aryl phosphates	Yasuda (1980)
Workplace air	automatic continuous air monitor using flame photometric detector	air monitor	0.12 mg/m^3	For air monitoring	Parker (1980)
Drinking-water	adsorb with XAD-2 resin, elute with acetone-hexane	GC/NPD GC/MS	1 ng/litre	method for low level trialkyl/aryl phosphates	Lebel et al. (1979, 1981)
River, sea and drinking-water	extract with methylene chloride or benzene	GC/NPD GC/FPD GC/MS	50 ng/litre	simultaneous method for trialkyl/aryl phosphates	Kenmotsu et al. (1980a, 1981, 1982) Ishikawa et al. (1985)
Waste water	extract with chloroform and separate with silica gel plate	TLC	2.5 mg/litre		Komlev et al. (1979)
River and sea sediment	extract with acetonitrile or acetone, clean up with charcoal or Florisil column chromatography	GC/FPD GC/MS	I ng/g	simultaneous method for trialkyl/aryl phosphates	Kenmotsu et al. (1980a, 1981, 1982) Ishikawa et al. (1985)
Fish	extract with acetonitrile and methylene chloride, clean up with acetonitrile-hexane partitioning, charcoal column chromatography, concentrated sulfuric acid extraction, and Florisil sulfuric column chromatography	GC/FPD GC/MS	1 ng/g	simultaneous method for trialkyl/aryl phosphates	Kenmotsu et al. (1980a)

17

Table 2 (contd).

Sample type	Sampling method extraction/clean-up	Analytical method[a]	Limit of detection	Comment	Reference
Fish	extract with acetone and hexane, clean up with acetonitrile-hexane partitioning and Florisil column chromatography	GC/FPD GC/NPD	10 ng/g	simultaneous method for organochlorine pesticides	EAJ (1977, 1978a,b)
Human adipose tissues	extract with benzene or acetone-hexane (15 + 85), clean up with gel permeation chromatography and Florisil column chromatography	GC/NPD GC/FPD GC/MS	1 ng/g	simultaneous method for trialkyl/aryl phosphates	Lebel & Williams (1983)

[a] NPD = nitrogen-phosphorous selective detector   FPD = flame photometric detector   GC = gas chromatography   TLC = thin-layer chromatography
   MS = mass spectrometry

adipose tissues. Gas-phase and particulate TBP in the atmosphere have been simultaneously collected on glycerol-coated Florisil® columns (Yasuda, 1980).

An octadecyl column has been used for extracting and concentrating TBP in blood plasma preparations (Pfeiffer, 1988). The sample was passed through the column from which TBP was eluted with chloroform. The recovery of 50 μg per litre was more than 90% of the TBP added to the column.

2.4.2 Clean-up procedure

Florisil column chromatography has been used for clean-up (Kenmotsu, et al., 1980a; Lebel & Williams, 1983; EAJ, 1984). This method allows the separation of TBP from other phosphate esters, e.g., TPP, and from organophosphorus pesticides, e.g., parathion. Sulfur-containing compounds, which often exist in sediment samples and interfere with the analysis of TBP by GC/FPD, are easily separated by elution with hexane from the Florisil column. Re-extraction with sulfuric acid from the hexane layer is a useful technique to avoid interference by sulfur-containing compounds (Kenmotsu et al., 1980a). However, it is difficult to separate TBP from lipids by Florisil column chromatography because of their similar polarities (Kenmotsu et al., 1980a). In such cases, gel permeation chromatography (GPC) is useful (where the elution volume varies depending on the type of phosphate ester, i.e. trialkyl, triaryl, or tri(haloalkyl) phosphates) (Lebel & Williams, 1983). Partitioning between acetonitrile and petroleum ether is an effective way of separating TBP from adipose tissue (Kenmotsu et al., 1980a; EAJ, 1984). Activated charcoal column chromatography has also been used to separate TBP from co-extractives of sediment samples (Kenmotsu et al., 1980a)

2.4.3 Gas chromatography and mass spectrometry

To identify TBP in environmental samples by packed column GLC, a comparison of each retention time using two types of liquid phase of different polarity is desirable. As a low polarity liquid phase, 3% or 10% OV-1 (Kenmotsu et al., 1980a; Ramsey & Lee, 1980), 2% or 3% SE-30 (Ramsey & Lee, 1980; EAJ, 1984), 2% or 3% OV-17 (Lebel et al., 1981; EAJ, 1984), 3% or 7% OV-101 (Sasaki et al., 1981; Lebel et al., 1981), SP-2100 (Rossum & Webb, 1978), 2% OV-225 (Yasuda, 1980), 2% DC-200 (EAJ, 1984), and 2% OV-17 plus 2% PZ-179 (Ishikawa et al., 1985) have been used. For the higher polarity liquid phase, 1% or 2% QF-1 (Bloom, 1973; Kurosaki et al., 1983), 5% FFAP, and 5% Thermon-3000 (Kenmotsu et al., 1980a, 1982) have been used. When a non-polar liquid phase is used in packed column GC, the reproducibility of the phosphate ester chromatogram is often poor. High loading of the liquid phase generally gives a good reproducibility (Kenmotsu et al., 1980a; Nakamura et al., 1980).

Capillary column GC has also been used for the identification and determination of TBP in environmental samples. Lebel et al. (1981) and Hutchins et al. (1983) used SP-2100 fused silica capillary column (25 m long; 0.22 mm internal diameter) for the determination of TBP in water samples. A wide-bore capillary glass column (25 m long) coated with OV-101 was used by Rogers & Mahood (1982).

Lebel & Williams (1983) used GC-MS for identifying TBP. The selected ion monitoring (SIM) technique is also useful for the quantification of low TBP levels (Lebel et al., 1981; Lebel & Williams, 1983; Ishikawa et al., 1985).

2.4.4 Contamination of analytical reagents

The widespread use of TBP in the plastics and paper industries may cause contamination of analytical reagents. Traces of TBP have been found in cyclohexane (Bowers et al., 1981; Karasek et al., 1981), methylene chloride (Lebel et al., 1981), activated charcoal, and Avicel (crystalline cellulose) (Kenmotsu et al., 1980a). Therefore, care must be taken in order to obtain reliable data in trace analysis of TBP.

2.4.5 Other analytical methods

TLC has been used for determining TBP. Bloom (1973) reported good separation of TBP by coupling TLC with GC. Komlev et al. (1979) described an analytical method for TBP in waste water and air using TLC. Tittarelli &

Mascherpa (1981) described a highly specific HPLC detector for TAPs using a graphite furnace atomic absorption spectrometer. In general, TLC and HPLC have not been as widely used as GC. Parker (1980) described the automatic monitoring of air using a flame photometric detector.

3. SOURCES OF HUMAN AND ENVIRONMENTAL EXPOSURE

3.1 Productions and processes

TBP does not occur naturally in the environment. Figures concerning total world production are not available. In Japan, 230 tonnes were produced in 1984[a], and 45 tonnes were produced in the USA in 1982 (Schultz et al., 1984). The estimated 1985 worldwide production capacity was 2720-4080 tonnes per year (US EPA, 1987a).

TBP is prepared by the reaction of phosphorus oxychloride with *n*-butanol (Windholz, 1983).

3.2 Uses

TBP is used as a solvent for cellulose esters, lacquers, and natural gums, as a primary plasticizer in the manufacture of plastics and vinyl resins, and as an antifoam agent (Sandmeyer & Kirwin, 1981; Windholz, 1983). In recent years, there has been a considerable increase in the use of TBP as an extractant in the dissolution process in conventional nuclear fuel processing (Parker, 1980; Laham et al., 1984; Schultz et al., 1984) and in the preparation of purified phosphoric acid (wet phosphoric acid method) (Davister & Peeterbroeck, 1982). Some 40% to 60% of all TBP consumed (probably in the USA) is used as a base stock in the formulation of fire-resistant aircraft hydraulic fluids (US EPA, 1985). In Japan, 140 tonnes was used in 1984 as an antifoaming agent (mainly in paper manufacturing plants), 40 tonnes as a metal extractant, and 50 tonnes for miscellaneous purposes[a]. TBP is also used as a constituent of cotton defoliants, which act by producing leaf scorching (Harris & May-Brown, 1976).

---

[a] Personal communication to IPCS from the Association of the Plasticizer Industry of Japan (1985)

4. ENVIRONMENTAL TRANSPORT, DISTRIBUTION, AND TRANSFORMATION

Summary

TBP has been found widely in environmental media (air, water, sediment, and biological tissues) but usually at low concentrations. Sources of TBP in the environment include leakage from sites of production and use (e.g., aircraft hydraulic fluids) and release from plastics or other products. No figures on the amounts released into the environment are available.

Once in the environment, it appears that the majority of TBP finds its way to sediments. Biodegradation in water is dependent on water quality (1 mg/litre was degraded in 7 days in River Mississippi water). Little or no degradation occurs in sterile river water or natural sea water. The degradation pathway most probably involves stepwise enzymatic hydrolysis.

In drinking-water treatment, TBP levels do not decrease unless powdered activated carbon is used, when very effective adsorption occurs (90-100% at a TBP concentration of 0.1 g per litre).

The bioaccumulation potential for TBP in killifish and goldfish is low, the bioconcentration factor ranging from 6 to 49. Depuration is rapid (half-life, 1.25 h).

There is no information on the fate of TBP in air, but this does not appear to be an area of concern. In addition, there are no data on transport to ground water.

4.1 Transport and transformation in the environment

4.1.1 Release to the environment

A major potential pathway of entry of TBP into the environment is by leakage from sites of production or use, and leaching from plastics disposed in landfill sites or aquatic environments. TBP has been found widely in air, water, sediment, fish, and several biota, but usually at low concentrations.

Extraction reagents and solvents are continuously lost from solvent extraction processes and may be transferred to aquatic environments. Ashbrook (1973), Ritcey et al. (1974), and Ashbrook et al. (1979) estimated the losses from solvent extraction plants. When recycled acid is used in the dissolution process in a conventional nuclear fuel reprocessing plant, TBP and its phosphate derivatives build up to a level where low concentrations of organophosphate vapour are released to the off-gas stream (Parker, 1980). However, no data on TBP levels in air at these plants are available.

TBP used in antifoaming agents may be lost from manufacturing plants into the environment, but the resultant amounts in the environment have not been measured. High concentrations of TBP have been detected in river water (7.61-25.2 μg/litre), fish (4.2-111.0 ng/g), and air over the sea (13.4 ng/m^3) sampled near Kawanoe City, Japan, where there are many paper manufacturing sites (Yasuda, 1980; Tatsukawa et al., 1975) (Table 5).

4.1.2 Fate in water and sediment

The solubility of TBP in water is considerably less than 1 g/litre at ambient temperatures (Table 1). Monitoring studies have shown that it is widely present in water and sediment (Suffet et al., 1980; Hattori et al., 1981; Williams & Lebel, 1981; Shinohara et al., 1981; Williams et al., 1982; Ellis et al., 1982; Kurosaki et al., 1983). The difference in TBP concentrations between water and sediment was estimated to be about 3 orders of magnitude (river water, 20-110 ng/litre; river sediment, 8-130 ng/g; sea water, 6-150 ng/litre; sea sediment, 2-240 ng/g) (EAJ, 1978a,b). The concentration factor of TBP on marine sediment was reported to be 4.3 (Kenmotsu et al., 1980b).

4.1.3 Biodegradation

The biodegradation of TBP in river water is slower than that of triphenyl phosphate and may depend to a considerable extent on water quality. Hattori et al. (1981) reported that 1 mg/litre completely disappeared in 6 days in Oh River water, Osaka, Japan, after a two-day lag period. However, at an initial TBP concentration of 20 mg per litre, only 21.9% was biodegraded in Oh River water after 14 days (Hattori et al., 1981). In Neya River water, Osaka, Japan, degradation started at 6 days and was complete after 9 days. In River Mississippi water (St. Louis waterfront, USA), degradation of TBP (1 mg/litre) started after 2 days and was complete within 7 days (Saeger et al., 1979). No degradation was observed in sterile river water (Saeger et al., 1979; Hattori et al., 1981) or in clear non-sterile sea water after 15 days (Hattori et al., 1981). Primary biodegradation rates from semicontinuous activated sludge studies (US Soap and Detergent Assoc., 1965; Mausner et al., 1969) generally showed the same trend in degradation rates as river die-away studies. TBP degradation was 96% complete at a 3-mg per litre, 24-h feed level, but only 56% (± 21%) at a 13-mg/litre, 24-h feed level (Saeger et al., 1979). The ultimate biodegradability of the phosphate esters was measured by Saeger et al. (1979) using the apparatus and procedure developed by Thompson & Duthie (1968) and modified by Sturm (1973). Two widely different results were obtained for the degradation TBP (20 mg/litre): 3.3% and 90.8% of the theoretical carbon dioxide evolution were measured in two experiments. Such differences are probably due to variations in the composite seed used in the two tests. A difference in the ratio of TBP to active biomass may have resulted in inhibition in the first case but not in the second (Saeger, et al., 1979).

The degradation pathway for TBP most likely involves stepwise enzymatic hydrolysis to orthophosphate and alcohol moieties (Pickard, et al., 1975). The alcohol would then be expected to undergo further degradation.

4.1.4 Water treatment

Fukushima and Kawai (1986) reported that 0.105-21.2 μg TBP/litre (geometric mean: 0.543 μg/litre) in untreated water was reduced to 0.018-3.80 μg/litre (geometric mean: 0.156 μg/litre) by conventional waste water treatment.

Piet et al. (1981) investigated the behaviour of organic compounds in dune infiltration: no change of concentration of TBP was observed. Sheldon & Hites (1979) reported that a TBP level of 400 ng/litre was not decreased by standard techniques for drinking-water treatment.

However, TBP is effectively adsorbed to powdered activated carbon (90-100% at a TBP concentration of 0.1 g/litre). The adsorption coefficient (Freundlich equation) obtained from an experiment using 0.01 to 10 mg TBP/litre at 25 °C was 190 (Ishikawa et al., 1985).

4.2 Bioaccumulation and biomagnification

Data reported on the bioaccumulation and depuration of TBP in killifish and goldfish are given in Table 3. No data for other fish species are available. Calculations of bioconcentration factors (BCF) for other species have been made on the basis of physico-chemical properties (Sasaki et al., 1981, 1982). However, these must be considered less reliable than the low values actually measured in killifish and goldfish.

Table 3. Bioaccumulation and clearance of TBP by fish

Species	Temp. (°C)	Flow/ stat	Bioconcen- tration factor[a]	Exposure conc. (mg/litre)	Depuration half life (h)	Reference
Killifish	25	stat	11-49	0.2-0.06		Sasaki et al. (1982)
(*Oryzias*		flow	16-27	0.84-0.1	1.25	
latipes)	25	stat	30-35	3-4		Sasaki et al. (1981)
Goldfish (*Carassius auratus*)	25	stat	6-11	3-4		Sasaki et al. (1982)

[a] Determined by GC-FPD

5. ENVIRONMENTAL LEVELS AND HUMAN EXPOSURE

Summary

TBP has been found frequently in environmental samples (air, water, sediment, and fish) but usually at low levels. Measured ambient air concentrations range from non-detectable to 41.4 ng/m³; the higher levels occurring near manufacturing sites. Surface water levels up to 25 200 ng/litre have been reported, but no groundwater sampling data are available. Levels in sediment range from 1 to 350 ng/g.

TBP levels in biological samples, including fish and shellfish, of up to 111 ng/g have been measured. It has also been detected in bird populations.

Human adipose tissues obtained from the autopsy of individuals with no known occupational exposure to TBP showed one positive sample (9.0 ng TBP/g) out of 16.

Exposure of the general population can occur by several routes, including the ingestion of contaminated drinking-water (levels up to 29.5 ng/litre), fish and shellfish, and other foodstuffs. US FDA total-diet studies have found average intake levels of 38.9, 27.7, and 2.7-6.2 ng/kg body weight per day for infants, toddlers, and adults, respectively.

Occupational exposure can occur in several industries, and especially where aircraft maintenance workers handle hydraulic fluids. Exposure during the synthesis of TBP and in plastics production is unlikely if protective measures are taken and because the various processes have been automated to a considerable extent.

Although production amounts are lower than for other triaryl/alkyl phosphates, TBP has been found frequently in environmental samples (water, sediment, and fish), whereas other triaryl/alkyl phosphates occur more rarely. However, the measured concentrations are usually low. These are listed in Tables 4-6.

Table 4. Concentration of TBP in air, water, and fish sampled in Northern Shikoku, Japan

Location	Date	Sample	Concentration[a]	Reference
Hiuchi-Nada area Hiuchi-Nada Sea (along Kannonji-Kawanoe)	1977, July	air	13.4 ng/m³	Yasuda (1980)
Other sampling areas on Seto Inland Sea	1977, June	air	2.3-3.5 ng/m³ (3/3)	Tatsukawa et al. (1975)
Kinsel River (Kawanoe City)	1974, July Nov. Dec.	water	7610 ng/litre 24 100 ng/litre 25 200 ng/litre	
Kawanoe Harbour	1974, Dec.	flatfish muscle, goby viscera	19.3 ng/g 111.0 ng/g	
Hatoba Harbour	1974	goby viscera, goby muscle	4.3 ng/g 4.2 ng/g	
Dogo Plain, Ozu Basin area Omoto River, Kutani River, etc.	1974	water	ND-187 ng/litre (4/10)	Tatsukawa et al. (1975)
Kawauchi Town	1976, July 1 Sep. 16 Sep. 17 Sep. 19 Sep. 20 Sep. 22 Nov. 18	air	3.1 ng/m³ 9.3 ng/m³ 6.1 ng/m³ 41.4 ng/m³ 25.7 ng/m³ 27.5 ng/m³ ND	Yasuda (1980)
Other locations	1976, July-Nov.	air	ND-6.4 ng/m³ (10/12)	

[a] Figures in parentheses indicate number of samples (detected/analysed); ND = not detected.

Table 5. Concentration of TBP in water, sediment, and fish at various locations

Year	Location	Sample	Concentration[a]	Number of samples (detected/analysed)	Reference
1973	Zurich (Switzerland)	lake water	54-82 ng/litre	2/2	Grob & Grob (1974)
		ground water	10 ng/litre	1/1	
		tap water	14 ng/litre	1/1	
1975	Japan (Various locations)	river and sea water	20-710 ng/litre	16/100	EAJ (1977)
		river and sea sediment	1-350 ng/g	34/100	
		fish	3-26 ng/g	31/94	
1977	Japan (Various locations)	river and sea water	6-580 ng/litre	39/117	EAJ (1978a,b)
		river and sea sediment	1.9-240 ng/g	48/117	
		fish	1.1-9.3 ng/g	27/85	
1976	Osaka (Japan)	river water	20-4500 ng/litre	12/13	Kawai et al. (1978)
1978	Eastern Ontario (Canada)	drinking-water	0.6-11.8 ng/litre	12/12	Lebel et al. (1981)
1978	Tokyo (Japan)	river water	60-2100 ng/litre	12/12	Wakabayashi (1980)
		sea water	50-870 ng/g	2/3	
		river sediment	0.9-7.7 ng/g	13/15	
		sea sediment	1.7-2.6 ng/g	3/3	
1979	Canada (Various locations)	drinking-water	0.2-62.0 ng/litre	57/60	Williams & Lebel (1981)
1979	River Nitelva (Norway)	river water	100-900 ng/litre	3/7	Schou & Krane (1981)
1980	Seto Inland Sea (Japan)	fish and shell fish	ND (2 ng/g)	0/41	Kenmotsu et al. (1981)

Table 5 (contd).

Year	Location	Sample	Concentration[a]	Number of samples (detected/analysed)	Reference
1980	Great Lakes (Canada)	drinking-water	0.8-29.5 ng/litre	24/24	Williams et al. (1982)
1980	Kitakyushu City (Japan)	river water	5-36 ng/litre	8/16	Ishikawa et al. (1985)
		sea water	ND (5 ng/litre)	0/9	
		sea sediment	ND (2 ng/g)	0/6	
1982	Niigata City (Japan)	river water	140 ng/litre	1/1	Kurosaki et al. (1983)
not reported	USA	city water	ND (50-500 ng/litre)	2/10	Muir (1984)

[a] ND = not detected; figures in parentheses indicate the limit of detection.

Table 6. Monitoring of TBP in wildlife performed by the Environmental Agency of Japan[a]

Year	Animal/species[b]	Location[c]	Concentration[d] (ng/g)	Number of samples (detected/analysed)
1980	Fish	various locations	ND	0/50
	Shellfish	various locations	ND	0/15
1981	Fish			
	Greenling	Yamada Bay	20	5/5
	Sea bass	Osaka Bay	Trace	5/5
	Other fish	various locations	ND	0/35
	Shellfish			
	Common mussel	Yamada Bay	10-20	5/5
	Other shellfish	various locations	ND	0/15
	Birds			
	Gray starling	Morioka	50-170	7/7
1982	Fish			
	Sea bass	Seto Inland Sea	10-20	2/5
	Other fish	various locations	ND	0/45
	Shellfish		ND	0/20
	Birds			
	Gray starling	Morioka	20-30	3/5
	Black-tailed gull	Tokyo Bay	ND	0/4

Table 6 (contd).

Year	Animal/species[b]	Locations[c]	Concentration[d] (ng/g)	Number of samples (detected/analysed)
1983	Fish	various locations	ND	0/50
	Shellfish	various locations	ND	0/20
	Birds			
	Gray starling	Morioka	30-250	5/5
	Black-tailed gull	Tokyo Bay	ND	0/5

[a] From : EAJ (1981, 1982, 1983, 1984)
[b] Monitoring species - Fish : chum salmon; angry rockfish; greenling; Pacific saury; cod; sea bass; dace
   - Shellfish : common mussel, Asiatic mussel
   - Bird : gray starling, black-tailed gull
[c] Monitoring locations :off the coast of Kushiro; off the coast of Nemuro (Hokkaido); Yamada Bay (Iwate);
   off the coast of Joban (Ibaraki); off the coast of Tohoku (Yamagata): Tokyo Bay; Osaka Bay;
   off the coast of Sanin (Tottori); Lake Eiwa (Shiga); Miura Peninsula (Kanagawa);
   Noto Peninsula (Ishikawa); Naruto (Tokushima)
[d] ND = not detected; detection limit = 10 ng/g

5.1 Environmental levels

5.1.1 Air

Yasuda (1980) investigated the distribution of various organic phosphorus compounds in the atmosphere above the Dogo Plain and Ozu Basin agricultural areas of Western Shikoku and above the Eastern Seto Inland Sea, Japan (Table 4). TBP concentrations were usually less than 10 ng per m^3, but higher concentrations (13.4-41.4 ng/m^3) were occasionally found. These higher atmospheric concentrations of TBP are probably due to fumes liberated from paper manufacturing plants located around Kawanoe City. However, the source of these higher concentrations has not been clearly identified. TBP has also been detected in the atmosphere in Okayama City, Japan, but the levels were less than 1 ng/m^3 (Kenmotsu et al., 1981).

5.1.2 Water

TBP has been widely detected in river, lake, and sea water in Europe, Japan, Canada, and the USA (Tables 4 and 5).

Tatsukawa et al. (1975) measured the distribution of five phosphate esters in river water in the Seto Inland Sea area of Japan and found 10 to several hundred ng per litre. Higher TBP concentrations (7600 to 25 200 ng/litre) were detected in Kinsei River, Kawanoe City, Japan. The authors suggested that these high concentrations were the result of effluent from paper manufacturing plants.

5.1.3 Sediment

Despite low sediment adsorption coefficients, TBP has frequently been detected in sediment samples in Japan (EAJ, 1978a,b; Wakabayashi, 1980; Rogers & Mahood, 1982; Ishikawa et al., 1985). The concentrations ranged from 1 to 350 ng/g.

5.1.4 Fish, shellfish, and birds

Although bioconcentration factors are low (section 4.2), significant concentrations of TBP (ranging from 1 to

30 ng/g) have been found frequently in fish and shellfish (Tables 4-6). Tatsukawa et al. (1975) reported a high concentration (111 ng/g) in the organs of goby caught in Kawanoe harbour at the entrance to the Kinsei River, Japan (Table 4). Although no clear evidence was available, this may have been due to pollution by paper manufacturing plants located around Kawanoe City. Rogers & Mahood (1982) also found TBP in fish caught downstream from pulp mills and a sewage plant outfall, but the concentrations were not reported.

Reports of wildlife monitoring by the Environmental Agency of Japan (EAJ, 1982, 1983, 1984) indicated TBP levels of 20-250 ng/g in birds (Gray starlings).

5.2 General population exposure

5.2.1 Food

The presence of TBP in infant and toddler total-diet samples and in adult diet samples was studied by Gartrell et al. (1986a,b). These samples were collected between October 1980 and March 1982 during a survey made for the US Food and Drug Administration (FDA). Gunderson (1988) also investigated the presence of TBP in samples collected between April 1982 and April 1984 during FDA total diet studies. TBP was only found in approximately 2% of the samples, corresponding to average daily intakes of 38.9, 27.7, and 2.7-6.2 ng/kg body weight per day for infants, toddlers, and adults, respectively.

Gilbert et al. (1986) analysed composite total-diet samples (representative of 15 different commodity food types encompassing an average adult diet for each of eight regions in the United Kingdom) for the presence of trialkyl and triaryl phosphates. Of the food groups, offal, other animal products, and nuts consistently contained the highest levels, but the proportion of individual compounds in the different food groups varied. Trioctyl phosphate was the major component in the carcass meat, offal, and poultry groups, and there were significant amounts of TBP and TPP. Total phosphate intake was estimated to be between 0.08 and 0.16 mg per person per day.

5.2.2 Drinking-water

TBP has been monitored in drinking-water in Canada (Suffet et al., 1980; Lebel et al., 1981; Williams & Lebel, 1981; Williams et al., 1982), and the concentrations ranged from 0.2 to 29.5 ng/litre.

5.2.3 Human tissues

Lebel & Williams (1983) analysed phosphate esters in human adipose tissue and detected TBP (9.0 ng/g) in one of 16 autopsy samples from humans with no known occupational exposure to TBP. In a similar study carried out by the US EPA (1986), a trace amount of TBP was detected in one of 46 samples.

5.3 Occupational exposure

In its 1981-1983 National Occupational Exposure Survey (NOES), the National Institute for Occupational Safety and Health (NIOSH), USA, estimated that 12 111 workers in 6 industries and 13 occupations were potentially exposed to TBP. Not included in this survey were workers involved in aircraft maintenance. Due to manipulation of hydraulic fluids containing TBP, these workers represent the largest population occupationally exposed. In 1988, the Tributyl Phosphate Task Force (TBPTF) of the Synthetic Organic Chemical Manufacturers Association (SOCMA) estimated that approximately 45 000 aircraft workers, the greatest number of workers potentially exposed to TBP, are exposed once per week for 30 min to 2 h to hydraulic fluids containing TBP (US EPA, 1987b, 1989).

6. EFFECTS ON ORGANISMS IN THE ENVIRONMENT

Summary

TBP is moderately toxic to aquatic organisms, the 96-h LC_{50} being 2.2 mg/litre for Daphnia and 4.2-11.4 mg/litre for fish in static tests. No data on non-target plants are available, but since the compound is used in desiccant defoliants, some damage to plants adjacent to treated areas could be expected.

6.1 Unicellular algae, protozoa, and bacteria

Toxicity data of TBP for protozoa, algae, and bacteria are given in Table 7. The inhibitory concentrations (EC_0, EC_{50}, EC_{100}) of TBP for the multiplication of unicellular algae, protozoa, and bacteria have been estimated to lie within the range of 3.2-100 mg/litre.

6.2 Aquatic organisms

Data on the toxicity of TBP for aquatic organisms are given in Table 8.

There is little difference in sensitivity between the few species of fish that have been studied; 96-h LC_{50} values range from 4.2 to 11.8 mg/litre. It seems that embryo-larval stages are less sensitive than post-natal stages of the fish life-cycle, but since the test conditions used were not identical this has not been fully confirmed. A series of tests carried out at different temperatures with rainbow trout suggested that toxicity increases with increasing temperature (Dave et al., 1979).

In studies by Dave & Lidman (1978), rainbow trout did not show any obvious effects at water concentrations below 5.6 mg TBP/litre but behaved very calmly when trapped in a hand-net at a concentration of 1 mg/litre (all concentrations are nominal value). At 10 mg/litre, the fish started showing severe balance disturbances, which included highly atypical movements like darting, coiling swimming, and backward somersaults, but they recovered after 24-72 h at this concentration. On the other hand,

Table 7. Toxicity of TBP to protozoa, unicellular algae, and bacteria

Organism	Species	Temperature (°C)	Habitat[a]	Exposure	Concentration (mg/litre)	Effect	Reference
Protozoa	Entosiphon sulcatum	25	F	3 days	14	Inhibition of cell multiplication: EC_0	Bringmann (1975, 1978); Bringmann & Kühn (1977a, 1981)
	Uronema parduczi	25	F	20 h	21	Inhibition of cell multiplication: EC_0	Bringmann & Kühn (1980, 1981)
	Chilomonas paramacecium	20	F	2 days	42	Inhibition of cell multiplication: EC_0	Bringmann & Kühn (1980, 1981)
Cyanobacterium (blue-green alga)	Microcystis aeruginosa	27	F	8 days	4.1	Inhibition of cell multiplication: EC_0	Bringmann (1975)
Green alga	Chlorella emersonii	25	F	2 days	10-50	Inhibition of cell multiplication: EC_{50}	Dave et al. (1979)
Green alga	Scenedesmus quadricaudata	27	F	7 days	3.2	Inhibition of cell multiplication: EC_0	Bringmann (1975); Bringmann & Kühn (1979)
Algae	13 algal species	20	F	14 days	50	Inhibition of cell multiplication: EC_{100}	Blanck et al. (1984)
Bacteria	Thiobacillus ferrooxidans	35	S	0-90 min	218[b]	Inhibition of oxygen uptake; 64% of control	Torma & Itzkovitch (1976)
	Pseudomonas putida	25	S	16 h	> 100	Inhibition of cell multiplication: EC_0	Bringmann & Kühn (1977a); Bringmann & Kühn (1979, 1980)

[a] F = fresh water; s = sediment
[b] Total organic carbon content

Table 8. Toxicity of TBP to aquatic organisms

Organisms	Age/size	Temperature (°C)	pH	Stat/renewal	Hardness (mg/litre)	End-point or criteria used	Effect	Concentration (mg/litre)	Reference
Rainbow trout (*Salmo gairdneri*)	Fry; 0.15 g	5	7.0	stat	45		96-h LC_{50}	9.4	Dave et al. (1979)
	Fry; 0.15 g	10	7.0	stat	45		96-h LC_{50}	11.8	Dave et al. (1979)
	Fry; 0.15 g	15	7.0	stat	45		96-h LC_{50}	8.2	Dave et al. (1979)
	Fry; 0.15 g	20	7.0	stat	45		96-h LC_{50}	4.2	Dave et al. (1979)
	20 g	15 (± 1)	8.5 (7.0-9.4)	stat	43.4		96-h LC_{50}	5-9	Dave & Lidman (1978)
	Embryo-larva; 2 weeks before hatching	8 (± 1)	8.3	stat-renewal	100	Egg: turning white to yellowish; larva: no response to mechanical stimulation	50-day LC_{0}	8	Dave et al. (1981)
Killifish (*Oryzias latipes*)	0.1-0.2 g	25		stat			96-h LC_{50}	9.6	Sasaki et al. (1981)
Goldfish (*Carassius auratus*)	0.8-2.8 g	25		stat			96-h LC_{50}	8.8	Sasaki et al. (1981)
Zebra fish (*Brachydanio rerio*)	0.25 g	25	8.3 (7.3-8.5)	stat	100		96-h LC_{50}	11.4[a]	Dave et al. (1981)
	Embryo-larva; 5 h after fertilization	25	8.3	stat-renewal	100	Egg: turning opaque; larva: no response to mechanical stimulation	10-day LC_{0}	13.5[a]	Dave et al. (1981)

Table 8 (contd).

Species									Reference
Goldenorfe (*Leuciscus idusmelanotus*)	5-7 cm, 1.5 (± 0.3) g	20 (± 1)	7-8	stat	269 (± 54)		48-h LC_{50}	7.6	Juhnke & Lüdemann (1978)
Waterflea (*Daphnia magna*)	<24 h	20	8.0	stat	200	Immobilization	24-h EC_{50}	30 (25-36)	Bringmann & Kühn (1982)
	24 h	20-22	7.6-7.7	stat	286		24-h LC_{50}	33	Bringmann & Kühn (1977b)
Fathead minnow (*Pimephales promelas*)	1.20 g	17.0	7.4	stat	44		96-h LC_{50}	1-10	Mayer et al. (1986)

[a] Nominal value

the balance disturbances persisted until the end of the experiment at a concentration of 11.5 mg/litre. At 13.5 mg per litre, the fish were immobilized, lying on their sides at the bottom of the water, and some of them died.

6.3 Plants

TBP is used as a constituent of cotton defoliants, producing leaf scorching, and is associated with an increase in the rate of leaf drying (Harris & May-Brown, 1976). Kennedy et al. (1955) reported that TBP increases the drying rate of lucerne, resulting in excessive leaf loss.

TBP applied by spraying as an emulsion (at a rate equivalent to 0.25% of freshly harvested leaf/weight) doubled the drying rate of ryegrass leaves. Leaf respiration stopped and did not resume in the subsequent 4 days (Harris & May-Brown, 1976). TBP has been shown to damage the leaf surface and help herbicides penetrate bean leaves (Babiker & Dancan, 1975; Turner, 1972).

There is no information on the effects of TBP on non-target plants, even at concentrations designed to produce desiccation of crop plants.

6.4 Arachnids

No mortality was observed among two-spotted spider mites (*Tetranychus urticae*) fed TBP at a concentration of 2 g/kg (Penman & Osborne, 1976).

7. KINETICS AND METABOLISM

Summary

TBP is readily absorbed (> 50%) from the gastrointestinal tract in rats. Some absorption of TBP through the skin also occurs, although the extent of dermal absorption is difficult to quantify from the data available. No information is available on the absorption of TBP following inhalation, and there is no satisfactory information on the distribution of TBP or its metabolites following absorption. The metabolism of TBP is characterized by oxidation of the butyl moieties. Oxidized butyl groups are removed as glutathione conjugates and subsequently excreted as N-acetyl cysteine derivatives. TBP metabolites are excreted predominantly in the urine, although smaller amounts also appear in the faeces and expired air.

7.1 Absorption

No information is available on the absorption of TBP following inhalation. Substantial absorption from the gastrointestinal tract occurred in rats given a single oral dose of TBP (Suzuki et al., 1984a,b; Khalturin & Andryushkeeva, 1986). Suzuki et al. (1984b) reported that more than 50% of an orally administered dose of TBP was absorbed within 24 h. Dermal absorption of TBP has been demonstrated in pigs, and there was little difference in the rate of skin penetration between regions with or without hair follicles (Schanker, 1971). In vitro investigations on isolated human skin showed that TBP has a high penetrating capacity. The average maximum steady-state rate of penetration through isolated human skin is 6.7 x 10^{-4} μmol/cm^2 per min (Marzulli et al., 1965).

In a study by Sasaki et al. (1985), TBP was poorly absorbed in goldfish but readily absorbed in killifish.

7.2 Distribution

Little information is available on the distribution of TBP and its metabolites. Following single or repeated oral dosing in rats, TBP was detected in the gastrointestinal tract, blood, and liver (Khalturin & Andryushkeeva, 1986).

7.3 Metabolism

The metabolic transformation of TBP has been studied in male rats following oral or intraperitoneal administration of ^{14}C-labelled TBP (Suzuki et al., 1984a,b). The first stage in the metabolic process appeared to be oxidation, catalysed by cytochrome P-450-dependent mono-oxygenase, at the w or w-1 position on the butyl chains. The hydroxy groups generated at the w and w-1 positions were further oxidized to produce carboxylic acids and ketones, respectively (Suzuki et al., 1984b). Following these oxidations, the oxidized alkyl moieties were removed as glutathione conjugates, which were then excreted as N-acetyl cysteine derivatives (Suzuki et al., 1984a). It has been reported that TBP is also metabolized in rodents to butyl-n-cysteine (Jones, 1970). However, the presence of butyl-n-cysteine was refuted by Suzuki et al. (1984a). In the urine, the major phosphorus-containing metabolites are dibutyl hydrogen phosphate, butyl dihydrogen phosphate, and butyl bis(3-hydroxybutyl) phosphate as well as small amounts of the following phosphates: dibutyl 3-hyroxybutyl, butyl 2-hydroxybutyl hydrogen, butyl 3-hydroxybutyl hydrogen, butyl 3-carboxypropyl hydrogen, 3-carboxypropyl dibutyl, butyl 3-carboxypropyl 3-hydroxybutyl, butyl bis (3-carboxypropyl), and 3-hydroxybutyl dihydrogen (Suzuki et al., 1984b)

The rate of metabolism of TBP and the nature of the metabolites produced were determined in *in vitro* tests on rat liver homogenate. It was found that rat liver microsomal enzymes rapidly metabolized TBP in the presence of NADPH (within 30 min), but only slight metabolic breakdown (11%) occurred in the absence of added NADPH. Dibutyl(3-hydroxybutyl) phosphate was obtained as a metabolite in the first stage of the test. The extended incubation time in the second stage of the test yielded two further metabolites, butyl di(3-hydroxybutyl) phosphate and dibutyl hydrogen phosphate, which were produced from the primary metabolite dibutyl(3-hydroxybutyl) phosphate (Sasaki et al., 1984). The degradation of TBP to these three metabolites has also been observed in *in vitro* studies on goldfish and killifish (Sasaki et al., 1985).

7.4 Excretion

In studies by Suzuki et al. (1984b), male Wistar rats (weighing 180-210 g) were given a single oral or intra-peritoneal dose of 14 mg ^{14}C-labelled TBP per kg body weight. Urine and faeces were collected separately. Within 24 h of oral administration, 50% of the radioac-tivity was eliminated in the urine, 10% in the exhaled air, and 6% in the faeces; the total elimination after 5 days was 82%. Following intraperitoneal injection, 70% of the radioactivity was eliminated in the urine, 7% by exhalation, and 4% in the faeces within 24 h; the total elimination after 5 days was 90%.

8. EFFECTS ON EXPERIMENTAL ANIMALS AND *IN VITRO* TEST SYSTEMS

Summary

Acute toxicity studies suggest that the chicken is the least sensitive species to TBP, rats and mice being more sensitive. A single injection of TBP produces clinical symptoms of mild anaesthesia, weakness, and respiratory failure.

Some short-term toxicity studies showed that TBP depresses body weight. However, other short-term studies showed no depression of body weight but histological evidence of degenerative changes in the seminiferous tubules. Further short-term studies indicated diffuse hyperplasia of the urinary bladder epithelium.

Mild to severe skin irritation, inducing erythema and oedema, has been reported together with mild irritation after instillation of TBP into the conjunctival sac of rabbits.

In mutagenicity studies, equivocal results have been obtained in the Ames test in the presence or absence of metabolic activation. However, Escherichia coli tests, Salmonella microsome tests, and recessive lethal mutation tests in Drosophila melanogaster all indicate that TBP is non-mutagenic.

TBP produces only mild plasma cholinesterase depression in rats. Short-term exposure results in the depression of caudal nerve conduction velocity and equivocal morphological changes in the Schwann cells of peripheral nerves.

Chicken dosed with high levels of TBP showed no evidence of ataxia or nerve and brain histopathology. These data demonstrate that TBP does not produce delayed neuropathy (i.e. OPIDN) in the chicken.

8.1 Single exposure

The acute lethality data for TBP are presented in Table 9.

Vandekar (1957) observed that a single injection of 80 or 100 mg TBP/kg in female rats produced clinical symptoms of mild anaesthesia, pronounced weakness, incoordination, and respiratory failure 1–2 h later.

Table 9. Acute lethality date for TBP

Species	Route of administration	LD_{50}/LC_{50} values	Reference
Rat	oral	1400 mg/kg	Johannsen et al. (1977)
	oral	1390-1530 mg/kg	Mitomo et al. (1980)
	oral	1552 mg/kg	Bayer AG (1986)
	oral	1600-3200 mg/kg	Eastman Kodak (1986)
	oral	3000 mg/kg	Dave & Lidman (1978)
	6-h inhalation	1359 mg/m^3	Eller (1937)
	intraperitoneal	800-1600 mg/kg	Eastman Kodak (1986)
	intravenous	100 mg/kg	Vandekar (1957)
Mouse	oral	900-1240 mg/kg	Mitomo et al. (1980)
	oral	400-800 mg/kg	Eastman Kodak (1986)
	intraperitoneal	100-200 mg/kg	Eastman Kodak (1986)
	subcutaneous	3000 mg/kg	Eller (1937)
Rabbit	dermal	> 3100 mg/kg	Johannsen et al. (1977)
Cat	4-5-h inhalation	2500 mg/m^3	Eller (1937)
Chicken	oral	1800 mg/kg	Johannsen et al. (1977)

Mitomo et al. (1980) reported acute toxicity studies on TBP. The oral LD_{50} values for ddY mice and Wistar rats were 1240 mg/kg (male mice), 900 mg/kg (female mice), 1390 mg/kg (male rats), and 1530 mg/kg (female rats).

8.2 Short-term exposure

In a short-term toxicity study with TCP and TBP, Wistar rats were fed pelleted diet containing a mixture of TBP and TCP at a concentration of 5000 mg/kg for 9 weeks (Oishi et al., 1982). The body weights of TBP-treated rats were significantly lower than those of the controls. Oishi and his co-workers also reported a short-term toxicity study with TBP in which Wistar male rats were fed diets containing 0, 5000 or 10 000 mg TBP/kg for 10 weeks (Oishi et al., 1980). The body weights and food consumption of the treated groups were significantly lower than those of the controls. The relative weights of the brain and kidneys in the high-dose group were significantly higher although the absolute weights were significantly lower than those of the control rats. Total protein and cholesterol in the high-dose group and blood urea nitrogen (BUN) in both TBP-treated groups were significantly higher than those in the controls. Cholinesterase activities were not inhibited. The blood coagulation time of the treated groups was significantly prolonged.

Laham et al. (1984) reported the results of a short-term toxicity study in which Sprague-Dawley rats were administered TBP by gavage at doses of 0.14 and 0.42 ml/kg for 14 days. No overt signs of toxicity were observed throughout the study. There were no significant differences in body weight between the test groups and their respective controls, but absolute and relative liver weights were significantly increased in the high-dose group (both sexes). Histopathological examination revealed a low incidence of degenerative changes in the seminiferous tubules of the high-dose group.

In a follow-up 18-week study, Laham et al. (1985) administered TBP by gavage once a day (5 days/week) to Sprague-Dawley rats (12 rats of each sex per group). Low-dose animals received 200 mg/kg per day throughout the study. High-dose animals received 300 mg/kg per day for the first 6 weeks and 350 mg/kg per day for the remaining 12 weeks. Histopathological examination of tissues revealed that all treated rats developed diffuse hyperplasia of the urinary bladder epithelium. Similar changes were not found in the control animals. No testicular changes were observed in the high-dose rats.

When Sprague-Dawley rats were fed diets containing TBP at levels of 0, 8, 40, 200, 1000, or 5000 mg/kg for 90 days, clinical chemistry changes included increased serum gamma-glutamyl transpeptidase levels in both sexes given 5000 mg/kg (Cascieri et al., 1985). Both absolute and relative liver weights were increased in both sexes at this dose. Histopathological studies indicated TBP-induced transitional cell hyperplasia in the urinary bladder of males given 1000 or 5000 mg/kg and females given 5000 mg per kg.

Mitomo et al. (1980) reported that seven consecutive daily oral intubations of TBP at doses of 140 or 200 mg per kg in Wistar rats resulted in marked increases in the relative weights of the liver and kidneys, increased BUN values, and tubular degeneration. The daily administration of 130 or 460 mg TBP/kg to rats for one month caused a marked depression of body weight gain and mortalities of 20 and 40%, respectively. Three-month feeding studies at TBP doses of 0, 500, 2000, or 10 000 mg/kg in ddY mice and SD rats produced dose-dependent depression of body weight gain accompanied by increases in liver, kidney, and testes weights and a decrease in uterine weight. Increased BUN values were found in the high-dose groups of both rats and mice.

8.3 Skin and eye irritation and skin sensitization

Smyth & Carpenter (1944) observed primary skin irritation effects following a single 0.01 ml application of TBP to the clipped belly of albino rabbits.

A single dermal application of 500 mg TBP to the intact or abraded skin of six rabbits produced severe irritation, inducing erythema and oedema in all the animals. The instillation of 100 mg TBP in the conjunctival sac of rabbits gave rise to mild irritation, which was noted 1, 2, 3, and 7 days following the application (FMC Corporation, 1985a).

A test on the irritating and corrosive potential of TBP, conducted according to the OECD Guidelines for Testing of Chemicals, No. 404 and 405 (OECD, 1981), showed that TBP was slightly irritating to rabbit skin (4-h exposure) and to rabbit eyes (Bayer AG, 1986).

Skin sensitization testing in human is inadequate (US EPA, 1987b, 1989). Although results suggest that TBP does not elicit any sensitization reaction in humans, the poor protocols used prevent any pertinent assessment.

8.4 Teratogenicity

Roger et al. (1969) reported that TBP was slightly teratogenic in chickens at high levels.

8.5 Mutagenicity and carcinogenicity

Hanna & Dyer (1975) reported that TBP was not mutagenic in recessive lethal mutation tests using *Drosophila melanogaster.* However, Gafieva & Chudin (1986) reported that TBP was mutagenic in the Ames test with Salmonella typhimurium TA 1535 and TA 1538 at concentrations of 500 and 1000 μg/plate both with and without metabolic activation. No mutagenicity was noted at lower concentrations (< 100 μg/plate).

The mutagenicity of TBP was also evaluated in S. typhimurium strains TA 98, TA 100, TA 1535 and TA 1538 (Ames Test) both in the presence and absence of added metabolic activation by Aroclor-induced rat liver S9 fraction. TBP, diluted with DMSO, was tested at concentrations up to 100 μl/plate using the plate incorporation technique. TBP did not produce a positive response in any strain with metabolic activation. Strains TA 1535, TA 1537, and TA 1538, without metabolic activation, produced twice the number of revertants per plate compared to the solvent control (DMSO) for at least three of the five test concentrations, but no dose-response relationship was observed (US EPA, 1978).

Tests on *Escherichia coli* strains WP2, WP2*uvr*A, CM561, CM571, CM611, WP67, and WP12 showed no mutagenic effect after 48 or 72 h of incubation at 37°C (Hanna & Dyer, 1975).

TBP was tested for mutagenic effects in a Salmonella/microsome test, both with and without S9 mix (metabolizing system), at doses of up to 12.5 mg/plate using four S. typhimurium LT2 mutants (histidine-auxotrophic strains TA 1535, TA 100, TA 1537 and TA 98). Doses of up to 120 μg/plate produced no bacteriotoxic effects. Bacterial counts remained unchanged. At high concentrations there was marked strain-specific bacterial toxicity so that only the range up to 500 μg/plate could be evaluated. There were no indications that TBP had any mutagenic effect (Bayer AG, 1985).

The testing of TBP at doses of 97 to 97 000 μg per plate, both with and without a metabolizing system (S9 mix), on S. typhimurium strains TA 98, TA 100, TA 1537, and TA 1538 confirmed the lack of mutagenic activity (FMC Corporation, 1985b).

No data are available on the carcinogenicity of TBP.

8.6 Neurotoxicity

Sabine & Hayes (1952) showed that both technical and reagent grades of TBP possess very weak cholinesterase activity and that very large doses produce cholinergic symptoms *in vivo*. They concluded that although TBP was capable of producing cholinergic symptoms, the doses required were so large that the "risk of accidental absorption of acutely toxic amounts is negligible. If the dosages for rats are roughly applicable to humans, it would be necessary for the development of symptoms that a human ingest a dose in the order of 100 ml or receive several millilitres parenterally". Sabine & Hayes (1952) found that TBP induced sleepiness and coma in male Sprague-Dawley rats when it was orally and parenterally administered.

Laham et al. (1983) reported the effects of TBP on the peripheral nervous system of Sprague-Dawley rats. In male rats fed TBP by gavage for 14 consecutive days (0.42 ml/kg per day) a small but significant reduction of caudal nerve conduction velocity, accompanied by morphological changes in the sciatic nerve, was found. Electron microscopic examination of sciatic nerve sections showed a retraction of Schwann cell processes in unmyelinated fibres, which may be interpreted as an early response to chemical insult. No axonal degeneration was observed in these animals. Laham et al. (1984) also investigated subacute oral toxicity of TBP in Sprague-Dawley rats and observed no overt signs of neurotoxicity (ataxia, convulsion, loss of righting reflex, etc.).

Johannsen et al. (1977) administered TBP orally to adult chickens at a cumulative dosage of 3680 mg/kg. No dysfunctional changes were noted during the period from 24 to 42 days following exposure. Formalin-fixed brain, sciatic nerve, and spinal cord samples examined 42 days after exposure showed no pathology.

9. EFFECTS ON HUMANS

Although there are no case reports of delayed neuro-toxicity resulting from TBP exposure, workers exposed to 15 mg TBP/m^3 air have complained of nausea and headaches (ACGIH, 1986).

TBP has a high capacity for skin penetration (Marzulli et al., 1965) and has been shown to have an irritant effect on the skin and mucous membranes in humans (Stauffer, 1984). It also appears to have an irritant effect on the eye and respiratory tract.

In an *in vitro* study, Sabine & Hayes (1952) found that TBP had a slight inhibitory effect on human plasma cholinesterase.

10. EVALUATION OF HUMAN HEALTH RISKS AND EFFECTS ON THE ENVIRONMENT

10.1 Evaluation of human health effects

There have been no reports that TBP has effects on occupationally exposed humans other than headache, nausea, and symptoms of skin, eye, and mucous membrane irritation. No cases of poisoning among the general population have been reported.

There is no indication from animal studies of a neurotoxic effect comparable to organophosphate-induced delayed neuropathy (OPIDN). Systemic toxicity in humans following acute exposure is likely to be low.

From *in vitro* test results, TBP is not considered to be mutagenic.

TBP is absorbed through the skin and so dermal exposure should be minimized.

The likelihood of long-term effects in occupationally exposed humans is small.

10.1.1 *Exposure levels*

The general population may be exposed to TBP through various environmental media, including drinking-water. However, the concentrations of TBP measured in drinking-water by the USA Environmental Protection Agency were extremely low and similar low levels were found in Japan, Canada, and Switzerland. Analyses in the USA of human adipose tissue revealed trace amounts of TBP in a small number of samples. There are insufficient data to evaluate the significance of general population exposure to TBP.

Workers involved in aircraft maintenance are potentially the most highly exposed population because of manipulation of hydraulic fluids containing TBP.

10.1.2 *Toxic effects*

Tributyl phosphate may enter the body by dermal penetration and by ingestion. However, the data available do not permit a useful comparison of the dermal and oral pharmacokinetics.

The available information does not permit an assessment of the risk presented by TBP as a potential carcinogen, neurotoxic agent, or dermal sensitizer. Observations relating to hyperplasia of urinary bladder epithelium in rats, neurotoxicity signs (ataxia, incoordination, weakness, respiratory failure) in rats, and sensitization of guinea-pigs are considered inadequate to evaluate the hazardous potential of TBP for human health. No tumour development has been observed in rats. TBP does not produce delayed neurotoxic effects in hens. No adequate data are available on the effects of TBP on reproduction (function of gonads, fertility, parturition, growth and development of offspring).

10.2 Evaluation of effects on the environment

Although, on the basis of physico-chemical properties, TBP has a high potential for bioaccumulation, measurements in laboratory experiments show that this is not realized in practice. Residues in biota sampled from the environment are generally low, though measurable residues in birds suggest that some transfer in the food chain is possible. Toxicity data are limited but suggest moderate toxicity to aquatic organisms. This information tends to support the view that TBP presents little risk to organisms in the environment since measured concentrations in surface waters are generally low.

10.2.1 Exposure levels

TBP has been found widely in surface water, sediment, and ground water, but normally only at low concentrations. The biodegradation of TBP in water is substantial under aerobic conditions but proceeds only at a slow rate below certain concentrations. It is possible that a low level equilibrium is reached in the environment between continuous release and removal. The lack of data on the rate of TBP hydrolysis does not permit a reliable assessment of the persistence of TBP in the environment. Consequently, the potential hazard of the substance cannot be evaluated. More data are required on the rate of TBP hydrolysis, which, when used with the available information on the biodegradability, will facilitate the assessment of its persistence and consequently the environmental risk posed by its manufacture, use, and disposal.

10.2.2 *Toxic effects*

The sensitivity of aquatic organisms to TBP has been determined in static tests. However, the biodegradability and relative hydrophobicity suggest that flow-through testing would provide more reliable data because of more constant exposure. The available information indicates moderate toxicity of TBP to algae, daphnids, and rainbow trout. TBP causes damage to terrestrial plants by increasing leaf drying rates, which results in excessive leaf loss. No information is available on uptake and translocation.

11. RECOMMENDATIONS

11.1 Recommendations for further research

There is a need for further studies on skin sensitization, teratogenicity and reproductive toxicity, and on the pharmacokinetics of different exposure routes.

Further testing for mutagenic potency is required. Initial *in vitro* tests on mammalian cell cultures should, if necessary, be followed by *in vivo* testing. Depending on the outcome of these mutagenicity tests, a carcinogenicity study may be required.

REFERENCES

ACGIH (1986) *Threshold limit values and biological exposure indices for 1986-1987,* Cincinnati, Ohio, American Conference of Governmental Industrial Hygienists.

ASHBROOK, A.W. (1973) A review of the use of carboxylic acids as extractants for separation of metals in commercial liquid-liquid extraction operations. *Miner. Sci. Eng., 5*: 169-180.

ASHBROOK, A.W., ITZKOVITCH, I.J., & SOWA, W. (1979) Losses of organic compounds in solvent extraction processes. In: *Proceedings of the International Solvent Extraction Conference (ISEC 77), Toronto, Canada, September 1977,* Toronto, Canadian Institute of Mining and Metallurgy, pp. 501-508 (CIM Special Vol. No. 21).

BABIKER, A.G.T. & DANCAN, H.J. (1975) Penetration of bean leaves by asulam as influenced by adjuvants and humidity. *Pestic. Sci.,* 6(6): 655-664.

BARNARD, P.W.C., BUNTON, C.A., LLEWELLYN, D.R., VERNON, C.A., & WELCH, V.A. (1961) The reactions of organic phosphates. Part V. The hydrolysis of triphenyl and trimethyl phosphates. *J. Chem. Soc.,* 1961: 2670-2676.

BAYER AG (1985) *[Tributyl phosphate: Salmonella/microsome test for investigation of point mutagenic effect],* Wuppertal, Bayer AG, Institute for Toxicology (Report No. 13805) (in German).

BAYER AG (1986) *[Tri-n-butyl phosphate: Studies on its irritation/corrosion potential for skin and eye rabbit (Report dated 26 March 1986) and: Studies on acute oral toxicity in male and female Wistar rats (Report dated 9 April 1986)],* Wuppertal, Bayer AG, Institute for Toxicology (in German).

BLANCK, H., WALLIN, G., & WANGBERG, S. (1984) Species-dependent variation in algal sensitivity to chemical compounds. *Ecotoxicol. environ. Saf.,* 8: 339-351.

BLOOM, P.J. (1973) Applications des chromatographies sur couche mince et gaz-liquide à l'analyse qualitative et quantitative des esters des acides phosphoriques et phosphoreux. *J. Chromatogr.,* 75: 261-269.

BOWERS, W.D., PARSONS, M.L., CLEMENT, R.E., EICEMAN, G.A., & KARASEK, F.W. (1981) Trace impurities in solvents commonly used for gas chromatographic analysis of environmental samples. *J. Chromatogr.,* 206: 279-288.

BRINGMANN, G. (1975) [Determination of the biological damaging action of water pollutants by the inhibition of the cell growth of the blue algae Microcystis.] *Gesund. Ing.,* 96(9): 238-241 (in German).

BRINGMANN, G. (1978) [Determination of the biological damaging action of water pollutants against protozoans.] *Z. Wasser Abwasser Forsch.*, 11: 210-215 (in German).

BRINGMANN, G. & KUHN, R. (1977a) [Limiting values for the damaging action of water pollutants to bacteria *(Pseudomonas putida)* and green algae *(Scenedesmus quadricauda)* in the cell multiplication inhibition test.] *Z. Wasser Abwasser Forsch.*, 10(3/4): 87-98 (in German).

BRINGMANN, G. & KUHN, R. (1977b) [Findings of the damaging action of water pollutants against *Daphnia magna.] Z. Wasser Abwasser Forsch.*, 10: 161-166 (in German).

BRINGMANN, G. & KUHN, R. (1979) [Comparison of the toxic limit concentrations of water pollutants against bacteria, algae and protozoans in the cell growth inhibitory test.] *Haustech. Bauphys. Umwelttech.*, 100(8): 249-252 (in German).

BRINGMANN, G. & KUHN, R. (1980) Comparison of the toxicity thresholds of water pollutants to bacteria, algae, and protozoans in the cell multiplication inhibition test. *Water Res.*, 14(3): 231-241.

BRINGMANN, G. & KUHN, R. (1981) [Comparison of the effect of harmful substances on flagellates and cilliates as well as on bacteriovorous and saprozoic protozoans.] *GWF Wasser Abwasser Gas- Wasserfach: Wasser/Abwasser*, 122(7): 308-313 (in German).

BRINGMANN, G. & KUHN, R (1982) [Results of toxic action of water pollutants on *Daphnia magna* tested by an improved standardized procedure.] *Z. Wasser Abwasser Forsch.*, 15(1): 1-6 (in German).

BRUNEAU, C., SOYER, N., BRAULT, A., & KERFANTO, M. (1981) Thermal degradation of tri-n-butyl phosphate. *J. anal. appl. Pyrolysis*, 3: 71-81.

CASCIERI, T., BALLESTER, E.J., SERMAN, L.R., MCCONNELL, R.F., THACKARA, J.W., & FLETCHER, M.J. (1985) Subchronic toxicity study with tributylphosphate in rats. *Toxicologist*, 5: 97.

DAVE, G. & LIDMAN, U. (1978) [Biological and toxicological effects of solvent extraction chemicals. Range finding acute toxicity in the rainbow trout and in the rat.] *Hydrometallurgy*, 3: 201-216 (in German).

DAVE, G., BLANCK, H., & GUSTAFSSON, K. (1979) Biological effects of solvent extraction chemicals on aquatic organisms. *J. Chem. Tech. Biotechnol.*, 29(4): 249-257.

DAVE, G., ANDERSSON, K., BERGLIND, R., & HASSELROT, B. (1981) Toxicity of eight solvent extraction chemicals and of cadmium to water fleas, *Daphnia magna*, rainbow trout, *Salmo gairdneri*, and zebrafish, *Brachydanio rerio. Comp. Biochem. Physiol.*, 69C: 83-98.

DAVISTER, A. & PEETERBROECK, M. (1982) The Prayon process for wet purification. *Chem. Eng. Prog.*, 78: 35-39.

EAJ (1977) *[Environmental monitoring of chemicals]*, Tokyo, Environment Agency Japan, pp. 212-214 (Environmental Survey Report Series, No. 3) (in Japanese).

EAJ (1978a) *[Environmental monitoring of chemicals]*, Tokyo, Environment Agency Japan, pp. 88, 94-96 (Environmental Survey Report Series, No. 4) (in Japanese).

EAJ (1978b) *Environmental monitoring of chemicals*, Tokyo, Environment Agency Japan, pp. 15, 21-22 (Environmental Survey Report of 1977 F.Y.).

EAJ (1982) *[Chemicals in the environment]*, Tokyo, Environment Agency Japan, pp. 95-97 (Office of Health Studies Report Series No. 8) (in Japanese).

EAJ (1983) *[Chemicals in the environment]*, Tokyo, Environment Agency Japan, pp. 96-101 (Office of Health Studies Report Series No. 9) (in Japanese).

EAJ (1984) *[Chemicals in the environment]*, Tokyo, Environment Agency Japan, pp. 106-111, 169-176 (Office of Health Studies Report Series, No. 10) (in Japanese).

EASTMAN KODAK (1986) *Summary of tributyl phosphate testing for acute toxicity, skin irritation, eye irritation and dermal sensitivity* (Submitted to US Environmental Protection Agency, Office of Toxic Substances, Washington DC) (TSCA 8(d) 062684(2)).

ELLER, H. (1937) *[The toxicology of technical plasticizers: Dissertation]*, University of Würzburg (in German).

ELLIS, D.D., JONE, C.M., LARSON, R.A., & SCHAEFFER, D.J. (1982) Organic constituents of mutagenic secondary effluents from wastewater treatment plants. *Arch. environ. Contam. Toxicol.*, 11: 373-382.

FMC CORPORATION (1985a) *Acute toxicity screening tests, Kronitex TBP: tributyl phosphate*, Philadelphia, Pennsylvania, FMC Corporation (Prepared for the US Environmental Protection Agency, Office of Toxic Substances, Washington DC) (Report FYI-OTS-0585-0380 FLWP).

FMC CORPORATION (1985b) *Kronitex TBP (tributyl phosphate) mutagenicity screening test, Salmonella microsomal assay (Ames test)*, Philadelphia, Pennsylvania, FMC Corporation (Prepared for the US Environmental Protection Agency, Office of Toxic Substances, Washington DC) (FYI-OTS-0585-0380 FLWP).

FUKUSHIMA, M. & KAWAI, S. (1986) [Present status and transition of selected organophosphoric acid triesters in the water area of Osaka city.] *Seitai Kagaku*, 8(4): 13-24 (in Japanese).

GAFIEVA, Z.A. & CHUDIN, V.A. (1986) [Evaluation of the mutagenic activity of tributyl phosphate on *Salmonella typhimurium*.] *Gig. i Sanit.*, 9: 81 (in Russian).

GARTRELL, M.J., CRAUN, J.C., PODREBARAC, D.S., & GUNDERSON, E.L. (1986a) Pesticides, selected elements and other chemicals in infant and toddler total diet samples, October 1980 - March 1982. *J. Assoc. Off. Anal. Chem.*, 69(1): 123-145.

GARTRELL, M.J., CRAUN, J.C., PODREBARAC, D.S., & GUNDERSON, E.L. (1986b) Pesticides, selected elements and other chemicals in adult total diet samples, October 1980 - March 1982. *J. Assoc. Off. Anal. Chem.*, 69(1): 146-159.

GILBERT, J., SHEPHERD, M.J., WALLWORK, M.A., & SHARMAN, M. (1986) A survey of trialkyl and triaryl phosphates in the United Kingdom total diet samples. *Food Addit. Contam.*, 3(2): 113-122.

GROB, K. & GROB, G. (1974) Organic substances in potable water and in its precursor. Part II. Applications in the area of Zurich. *J. Chromatogr.*, 90: 303- 313.

GUNDERSON, E.L. (1988) FDA total diet study, April 1982 - April 1984, dietary intakes of pesticides, selected elements and other chemicals. *J. Assoc. Off. Anal. Chem.*, 71(6): 1200-1209.

HANNA, P.J. & DYER, K.F. (1975) Mutagenicity of organophosphorus compounds in bacteria and Drosophila. *Mutat. Res.*, 28: 405-420.

HARRIS, C.E. & MAY-BROWN, R. (1976) The effect of tri-n-butyl phosphate on the drying rate and respiration rate of grass leaves measured in the laboratory. *J. Agric. Sci. Camb.*, 86: 531-535.

HATTORI, Y., ISHIKAWA, H., KUGE, Y., & NAKAMOTO, M. (1981) [Environmental fate of organic phosphate esters.] *Suishitu Odaku Kenkyu*, 4: 137-141 (in Japanese).

HIGGINS, C.E., BALDWIN, W.H., & SOLDANO, B.A. (1959) Effects of electrolytes and temperature on the solubility of tributyl phosphate in water. *J. phys. Chem.*, 63: 113-118.

HUTCHINS, S.R., TOMSON, M.B., & WARD, C.H. (1983) Trace organic contamination of ground water from a rapid infiltration site: A laboratory-field coordinated study. *Environ. Toxicol. Chem.*, 2: 195-216.

ISHIKAWA, S., TAKETOMI, M., & SHINOHARA, R. (1985) Determination of trialkyl and triaryl phosphates in environmental samples. *Water Res.*, 19: 119-125.

JOHANNSEN, F.R., WRIGHT, P.L., GORDON, D.E., LEVINSKAS, Q.J., RADUE, R.W., & GRAHAM, P.R. (1977) Evaluation of delayed neurotoxicity and dose-response relationships of phosphate esters in the adult hen. *Toxicol. appl. Pharmacol.*, 41: 291-304.

JONES, A.R. (1970) Metabolism of trialkyl phosphates. *Experientia (Basel)*, 26: 492-493.

JUHNKE, I. & LUDEMANN, D. (1978) [The results obtained with the Golden Orfe test, during the examination of 200 selected chemical compounds, under comparable conditions in two different laboratories, are presented.] *Z. Wasser Abwasser Forsch.*, 11(5): 161-164 (in German).

KARASEK, F.W., CLEMENT, R.E., & SWEETMAN, J.A. (1981) Preconcentration for trace analysis of organic compounds. *Anal. Chem.*, 53(9): 1050A-1054A, 1056A-1058A.

KAWAI, S., FUKUSHIMA, M., ODA, K., & UNO, G. (1978) [Water pollution caused by organophosphoric compounds.] *Kankyo Gijyutsu*, 7: 668-675 (in Japanese).

KENMOTSU, K., MATSUNAGA, K., & ISHIDA, T. (1980a) [Multiresidue determination of phosphoric acid triesters in fish, sea sediment and sea water.] *J. Food Hyg. Soc. Jpn*, 21: 18-31 (in Japanese).

KENMOTSU, K., MATSUNAGA, K., & ISHIDA, T. (1980b) [Studies on the mechanisms of biological activities of various environmental pollutants. V: Environmental fate of organic phosphoric acid triesters.] *Okayamaken Kankyo Hoken Senta Nempo*, 4: 103-110 (in Japanese).

KENMOTSU, K., MATSUNAGA, K., SAITO, N., & OGINO, Y. (1981) [An environmental survey of chemicals. XVII. Multiresidue determination of organic phosphate esters in environment samples.] *Okayamaken Kankyo Hoken Senta Nempo*, 5: 145-156 (in Japanese).

KENMOTSU, K., MATSUNAGA, K., WAITO, N., OGINO, Y., & ISHIDA, T. (1982) [An environmental survey of chemicals. II: Determination of organo-phosphoric acid triesters.] *Okayamaken Kankyo Hoken Senta Nempo*, 6: 126-132 (in Japanese).

KENNEDY, V.K., HESSE, W.H., & JOHNSON, C.M. (1955) The effect of herbicides on the drying rate of hay crops. *Agron. J.*, 46: 199-203.

KHALTURIN, G.V. & ANDRYUSHKEEVA, N.I. (1986) Toxicokinetics of tributyl phosphate following single and chronic intragastric intake by rats. *Gig. i Sanit.*, 2: 87.

KOMLEV, I.V., DAKHNOV, P.P., & TROITSKABA, L.M. (1979) [Thin layer chromatographic determination of tributyl phosphate in waste water of chemical plant.] *Khim. Prom-st Ser. Metody Anal Kontrolya Kach Prod Khim Prom-sti.*, 5: 19-22 (in Russian).

KUROSAKI, H., TOMINAGA, Y., MUKAI, H., & OZAKI, K. (1983) [Trace analysis of pesticides in river water and sediment. III. Analytical method of organophosphorus pesticides in river water.] *Bull. environ. Pollut. Center Niigata*, 8: 70-74 (in Japanese).

LAHAM, S., SZABO, J., & LONG, G. (1983) Effects of tri-n-butyl phosphate on the peripheral nervous system of the Sprague-Dawley rat. *Drug chem. Toxicol.*, 6(4): 363-377.

LAHAM, S., LONG, G., & BROXUP, B. (1984) Subacute oral toxicity of tri-n-butyl phosphate in the Sprague-Dawley rat. *J. appl. Toxicol.*, 4: 150-154.

LAHAM, S., LONG, G., & BROXUP, B. (1985) Induction of urinary bladder hyperplasia in Sprague-Dawley rats orally administered tri-n-butyl phosphate. *Arch. environ. Health*, 40: 301-306.

LEBEL, G.L. & WILLIAMS, D.T. (1983) Determination of organic phosphate triesters in human adipose tissue. *J. Assoc. Off. Anal. Chem.*, 66: 691-699.

LEBEL, G.L., WILLIAMS, D.T., GRIFFITH, G., & BENOIT, F.M. (1979) Isolation and concentration of organophosphorus pesticides from drinking water at the ng/L level, using macroreticular resin. *J. Assoc. Off. Anal. Chem.*, 62: 241-249.

LEBEL, G.L., WILLIAMS, D.T., & BENOIT, F.M. (1981) Gas chromatographic determination of trialkyl/aryl phosphates in drinking water, following isolation using macroreticular resin. *J. Assoc. Off. Anal. Chem.*, 64: 991-998.

MARZULLI, F.N., CALLAHAN, J.F., & BROWN, D.W.C. (1965) Chemical structure and skin penetrating capacity of a short series of organic phosphates and phosphoric acid. *J. invest. Dermatol.*, 44: 339-344.

MAUSNER, M., BENEDICT, J.H., BOOMAN, K.A., BRENNER, T.E., CONWAY, R.A., DUTHIE, J.R., GARRISON, L.J., HENDRIX, C.D., & SHEWMAKER, J.E. (1969) The status of biodegradability testing of nonionic surfactants. *J. Am. Oil Chem. Soc.*, 46: 432-440.

MAYER, F.L., Jr, MAYER, K.S., & ELLERSIECK, M.R. (1986) Relation of survival to other endpoints in chronic toxicity tests with fish. *Environ. Toxicol. Chem.*, 5(8): 737-748.

MITOMO, T., ITO, T., UENO, Y., & TERAO, K. (1980) Toxicological studies on tributyl phosphate. I. Acute and subacute toxicities. *J. toxicol. Sci.*, 5: 270-271.

MODERN PLASTICS ENCYCLOPEDIA (1975) International Advertising Supplement 52 (10A), p. 697, New York, McGraw-Hill Inc.

MUIR, D.C.G. (1984) Phosphate esters. In: Hutzinger, O., ed. *The handbook of environmental chemistry*, Berlin, Heidelberg, New York, Tokyo, Springer-Verlag, Vol. 3, Part C, pp. 41-66.

NAKAMURA, A., KOJIMA, S., & KANIWA, M. (1980) Quantitative gas chromatographic determination of tris(2,3-dibromopropyl)phosphate in the 10-ng range by using a 0.8-mm I.D. column packed with a high liquid loaded support. *J. Chromatogr.*, 196: 133-141.

OECD (1981) *OECD guidelines for testing of chemicals. Section 2: Effects on biotic systems*, Paris, Organization for Economic Cooperation and Development, Publications Office.

OISHI, H., OISHI, S., & HIRAGA, K. (1980) Toxicity of tri-n-butyl phosphate, with special reference to organ weights, serum components and cholinesterase activity in male rats. *Toxicol. Lett.*, **6**: 81-85.

OISHI, H., OISHI, S., & HIRAGA, K. (1982) Toxicity of several phosphoric acid esters in rats. *Toxicol. Lett.*, **13**: 29-34.

PACIOREK, K.J.L., KRATZER, R.H., KAUFMAN, J., NAKAHARA, J.H., CHRISTOS, T., & HARTSTEIN, A.M. (1978) Thermal oxidative degradation studies of phosphate esters. *Am. Ind. Hyg. Assoc. J.*, **39**: 633-639.

PARKER, G.B. (1980) Continuous quantitative analysis of low concentrations of tributyl phosphate (TBP) vapors in flowing air streams. *Am. Ind. Hyg. Assoc. J.*, **41**: 220-222.

PENMAN, D.R. & OSBORNE, G.O. (1976) Trialkyl phosphates and related compounds as antifertility agents of the two-spotted spider mite. *J. econ. Entomol.*, **69**(2): 266-268.

PFEIFFER, P. (1988) [Determination of tri-n-butyl phosphate in plasma preparations using solid phase extraction and capillary gas chromatography.] *J. clin. Chem. clin. Biochem.*, **26**(4): 229-231 (in German).

PICKARD, M.A., WHELIHAN, J.A., & WESTLAKE, D.W.S. (1975) Utilization of triaryl phosphates by a mixed bacterial population. *Can. J. Microbiol.*, **21**: 140-145.

PIET, G.J., MORRA, C.H.F., & DE KRUIJF, H.A.M. (1981) The behaviour of organic micropollutants during passage through the soil. Quality of groundwater, Proceedings of an international symposium, Noordwijkerhout, The Netherlands. *Stud. environ. Sci.*, **17**: 557-564.

RAMSEY, J.D. & LEE, T.D. (1980) Gas-liquid chromatographic retention indices of 296 non-drug substances on SE-30 or OV-1 likely to be encountered in toxicological analyses. *J. Chromatogr.*, **184**: 185-206.

RITCEY, G.M., LUCAS, B.M., & ASHBROOK, A.W. (1974) Some comments on the loss, and environmental effects of solvent extraction reagents used in metallurgical processing. *Proc. Int. Solvent Extr. Conf.*, **3**: 2873-2884.

ROGER, J.-C., UPSHALL, D.G., & CASIDA, J.E. (1969) Structure-activity and metabolism studies on organophosphate teratogens and their alleviating agents in developing hen eggs with special emphasis on bidrin. *Biochem. Pharmacol.*, **18**: 373-392.

ROGERS, L.H. & MAHOOD, H.W. (1982) *Environmental monitoring of the Fraser River at Prince George. Chemical analysis of fish, sediment, municipal sewage and bleached kraft wastewater samples*, West Vancouver, British Columbia, Department of Fisheries and Oceans, West Vancouver Laboratory (Canadian Technical Report of Fisheries and Aquatic Science, No. 1135).

ROSSUM, P.V. & WEBB, R.G. (1978) Isolation of organic pollutants by XAD resins and carbon. *J. Chromatogr.*, **150**: 381-392.

SABINE, J.C. & HAYES, F.N. (1952) Anticholinesterase activity of tributyl phosphate. *Arch. ind. Hyg. occup. Med.*, **6**: 174-177.

SAEGER, V.W., HICKS, O., KALEY, R.G., MICHAEL, P.R., MIEURE, J.P., & TUCKER, E.S. (1979) Environmental fate of selected phosphate esters. *Environ. Sci. Technol.*, **13**: 840-844.

SANDMEYER, E.E. & KIRWIN, C.J. (1981) Esters. In: Clayton, G.D. & Clayton, F.E., ed. *Patty's industrial hygiene and toxicology*, 3rd revised ed., New York, Wiley-Interscience, Vol. 2A, pp. 2259-2412.

SASAKI, K., TAKEDA, M., & UCHIYAMA, M. (1981) Toxicity, absorption and elimination of phosphoric acid triesters by Killifish and Goldfish. *Bull. environ. Contam. Toxicol.*, **27**: 775-782.

SASAKI, K., SUZUKI, T., TAKEDA, M., & UCHIYAMA, M. (1982) Bioconcentration and excretion of phosphoric acid triesters by Killifish *(Oryzeas latipes)*. *Bull. environ. Contam. Toxicol.*, **28**: 752-759.

SASAKI, K., SUZUKI, T., TAKEDA, M., & UCHIYAMA, M. (1984) Metabolism of phosphoric acid triesters by rat liver homogenate. *Bull. environ. Contam. Toxicol.*, **33**: 281-288.

SASAKI, K., SUZUKI, T., TAKEDA, M., & UCHIYAMA, M. (1985) [Metabolism of phosphoric acid triesters by goldfish, *Carassius auratus*.] *Eisei Kagaku,* **31**(6): 397-404 (in Japanese).

SCHANKER, L.S. (1971) Drug absorption. In: La Du, B.N., Mandel, H.G., & Way, E.L., ed. *Fundamentals of drug metabolism and disposition,* Baltimore, Maryland, Williams and Wilkins, pp. 22-43.

SCHOU, L. & KRANE, J.E. (1981) Organic micropollutants in a Norwegian watercourse. *Sci. total Environ.*, **20**(30): 277-286.

SCHULTZ, W.W., NAVRATIL, J.D., & TALBOT, A.E. (1984) *Science and technology of tributyl phosphate Vol. 1, Synthesis, properties, reactions and analysis,* Boca Raton, Florida, CRC Press.

SHELDON, L.S. & HITES, R.A. (1979) Sources and movement of organic chemicals in the Delaware River. *Environ. Sci. Technol.*, **13**: 574-579.

SHINOHARA, R., KIDO, A., ETO, S., HORI, T., KOGA, M., & AKIYAMA, T. (1981) Identification and determination of trace organic substances in tap water by computerized gas chromatography-mass spectrometry and mass fragmentography. *Water Res.*, **15**: 535-542.

SMYTH, H.F. & CARPENTER, C.P. (1944) The place of the range finding test in the industrial toxicology laboratory. *J. ind. Hyg. Toxicol.*, **26**: 269-273.

STURM, R.N. (1973) Biodegradability of nonionic surfactants: Screening test for predicting rate and ultimate biodegradation. *J. Am. Oil Chem. Soc.*, **50**: 159-167.

SUFFET, I., BRENNER, L., & CAIRO, P.R. (1980) GC/MS identification of trace organics in Philadelphia drinking waters during a 2-year period. *Water Res.,* 14: 853-867.

SUZUKI, T., SASAKI, K., TAKEDA, M., & UCHIYAMA, M. (1984a) Some S-containing metabolites of tributyl phosphate in the rat. *J. agric. food Chem.,* 32: 1278-1283.

SUZUKI, T., SASAKI, K., TAKEDA, M., & UCHIYAMA, M. (1984b) Metabolism of tributyl phosphate in male rats. *J. agric. food Chem.,* 32: 603-610.

TATSUKAWA, R., WAKIMOTO, T., & OKADA, T. (1975) [Water pollution with organic phosphoric ester plasticizers and flame retardants.] *Nihon Suishitu Odaku Kenkyu Kyokai Symp. Ser.,* 9: 7-12 (in Japanese).

THOMPSON, J.E. & DUTHIE, J.R. (1968) Biodegradability and treatability of nitrilotriacetate. *Water Pollut. Control Fed.,* 40: 306-319.

TITTARELLI, P. & MASCHERPA, A. (1981) Liquid chromatography with graphite furnace atomic absorption spectophotometric detector for speciation of organophosphorous compounds. *Anal. Chem.,* 53: 1466-1469.

TORMA, A.E. & ITZKOVITCH, I. J. (1976) Influence of organic solvents on chalcopyrite oxidation ability of *Thiobacillus ferrooxidans. J. appl. environ. Microbiol.,* 10(2): 102-107.

TURNER, D.J. (1972) The influence of additives on the penetration of foliar applied growth regulator herbicides. *Pestic. Sci.,* 3: 323-331.

US EPA (1978) *Kronite TBP (tributyl phosphate) mutagenicity screening test Salmonella microsomal assay (Ames test),* Washington, DC, US Environmental Protection Agency, Office of Pesticides and Toxic Substances.

US EPA (1985) *Chemical hazard information profile draft report: tri(alkyl/ alkoxy) phosphates,* Washington, DC, US Environmental Protection Agency, Office of Toxic Substances.

US EPA (1986) *Broad scan analysis tissue survey specimens Volume III - Semi-volatile organic compounds,* Washington, DC, US Environmental Protection Agency, Office of Pesticides and Toxic Substances.

US EPA (1987a) *Aggregated production volume for CASRN 128-73-8, 1985,* Washington, DC, US Environmental Protection Agency, Confidential Data Branch, Office of Toxic Substances.

US EPA (1987b) Tributyl phosphate: Proposed test rule. *Fed. Reg.,* 52(218): 43346-43366.

US EPA (1989) Tributyl phosphate: Final test rule. *Fed. Reg.,* 54(155): 33400-33415.

US SOAP AND DETERGENT ASSOCIATION (1965) A procedure and standards for the determination of the biodegradability of alkyl benzene sulfonate and linear alkylate sulfonate (Report of the Subcommittee on Biodegradation Test Methods). *J. Am. Oil Chem. Soc.*, **42**: 986-993.

VANDEKAR, M. (1957) Anaesthetic effect produced by organophosphorus compounds. *Nature (Lond.)*, **179**: 154-155.

WAKABAYASHI, A. (1980) [Environmental pollution caused by organophosphoric fire-proofing plasticizers.] *Annu. Rep. Tokyo Metrop. Res. Inst Environ. Prot.*, **11**: 110-113 (in Japanese).

WILLIAMS, D.T. & LEBEL, G.L. (1981) A national survey of tri(haloalkyl)-, trialkyl-, and triarylphosphates in Canadian drinking water. *Bull. environ. Contam. Toxicol.*, **27**: 450-457.

WILLIAMS, D.T., NESTMANN, E.R., LEBEL, G.L., BENOIT, F.M., & OTSON, R. (1982) Determination of mutagenic potential and organic contaminants of Great Lakes drinking water. *Chemosphere*, **11**: 263-276.

WINDHOLZ, M., ed. (1983) *The Merck index*, 10th ed., Rahway, New Jersey, Merck and Co., Inc.

YASUDA, H. (1980) [Concentration of organic phosphorus pesticides in the atmosphere above the Dogo plain and Ozu basin.] *J. Chem. Soc. Jpn*, **4**: 645-653 (in Japanese).

RESUME

1. Identité, propriétés physiques et chimiques, méthodes d'analyse

Le phosphate de tri-*n*-butyle (TBP) est un liquide ininflammable, inexplosible, incolore et inodore. Toutefois, il est instable à la chaleur et commence à se décomposer à des températures inférieures à son point d'ébullition. Par analogie avec les propriétés chimiques du phosphate de triméthyle, il devrait subir une hydrolyse rapide en milieu acide neutre ou alcalin. C'est un agent faiblement alkylant. Son coefficient de partage entre l'octanol et l'eau (log de P_{ow}) est de 3,99-4,01.

Pour l'analyse, la méthode choix est la chromatographie gaz-liquide, avec détection au moyen d'un dispositif sensible à l'azote/phosphore ou par photométrie de flamme. Les réactifs pour analyse sont fréquemment contaminés par du TBP; aussi, faut-il veiller à ce problème lorsqu'on s'efforce d'obtenir des données fiables sur la recherche de traces de TBP.

2. Sources d'exposition humaine et environnementale

Le phosphate de tri-*n*-butyle est produit par réaction du *n*-butanol sur l'oxychlorure de phosphore. On l'utilise comme solvant des esters cellulosiques, des vernis et des gommes naturelles et comme plastifiant pour différentes matières plastiques, notamment les résines vinyliques. On l'utilise également pour l'extraction des métaux, comme base dans la préparation des liquides hydrauliques ininflammables destinés à l'aéronautique et comme agent antimousse. Au cours des dernières années, l'usage du TBP comme solvant d'extraction dans le procédé par dissolution utilisé pour le retraitement du combustible nucléaire, s'est beaucoup développé.

On peut considérer qu'en utilisation normale, la population dans son ensemble n'encourt qu'une exposition minime.

3. Transport, distribution et transformation dans l'environnement

Lorsqu'on l'utilise comme réactif, comme solvant d'extraction ou comme agent antimousse, le TBP s'échappe continuellement dans l'atmosphère et dans le milieu aquatique. Sa biodégradation est moyennement lente à lente selon sa proportion par rapport à la biomasse active. Elle comporte une hydrolyse enzymatique en plusieurs étapes conduisant à un orthophosphate et au *n*-butanol, lequel est dégradé à son tour. Les techniques ordinaires de traitement de l'eau de consommation ne réduisent pas sa teneur en phosphate de tributyle.

Les facteurs de bioconcentration mesurés chez deux espèces de poissons (un cyprinodontidé et le poisson rouge) vont de 6 à 49. La demi-vie d'élimination est de 1,25 heure chez ces poissons.

4. Niveaux dans l'environnement et exposition humaine

On trouve fréquemment du TBP dans l'air, l'eau, les sédiments et les organismes aquatiques mais les prélèvements effectués n'en contiennent que de faibles quantités. On en a trouvé de plus fortes concentrations dans l'air, l'eau et les poissons prélevés à proximité d'usines de pâte à papier au Japon: 13,4 ng/m^3 dans l'air, 25 200 ng par litre dans l'eau de rivière et 111 ng/gramme dans les organes pisciaires. Des études de ration totale effectuées au Royaume-Uni et aux Etats-Unis indiquent que l'apport alimentaire moyen quotidien de TBP est d'environ 0,02 à 0,08 μg/kg de poids corporel.

5. Effets sur les êtres vivants dans leur milieu naturel

On estime que la concentration inhibant la multiplication des algues unicellulaires, des protozoaires et des bactéries (CE_0, CE_{50}, CE_{100}), se situe dans les limites de 3,2 à 100 mg/litre. La toxicité aiguë pour les poissons (CL_{50}) varie de 4,2 à 11,8 mg/litre. Le TBP augmente la vitesse de dessèchement des feuilles, entraînant une inhibition rapide et complète de la respiration foliaire.

6. Cinétique et métabolisme

Administré par voie orale ou injecté par voie intrapéritonéale à des animaux de laboratoire, le TBP est rapidement transformé par le foie et peut-être aussi par le rein en produits d'hydroxylation au niveau des restes butyliques. Le TBP est principalement excrété sous la forme d'hydrogénophosphate de dibutyle, de dihydrogéno-phosphate de butyle et de phosphate de butyle et de bis-hydroxy-3 butyle. Les restes alkyles hydroxylés sont éliminés et excrétés sous forme de N-acétylalkyl cystéine et de gaz carbonique.

7. Effets sur les animaux d'expérience et les systèmes d'épreuve *in vitro*

Les valeurs de la DL_{50} par voie orale chez la souris et le rat seraient d'environ 1 à 3 g/kg ce qui indique une toxicité aiguë relativement faible.

Des études de toxicité subchronique ont permis d'observer une réduction du gain de poids liée à la dose ainsi qu'une augmentation du poids du foie, des reins et des testicules. Le rein semble être l'organe cible du phosphate de tri-n-butyle.

L'irritation cutanée provoquée par le TBP chez des lapins albinos paraît aussi sévère qu'avec la morpholine.

Le TBP serait légèrement tératogène à fortes doses. Quant à son pouvoir mutagène, il n'a pas été suffisamment étudié. Des résultats négatifs ont été signalés à la suite d'épreuves sur bactéries ainsi qu'après une épreuve de mutation létale récessive sur *Drosophila melanogaster*.

Il n'existe pas de données suffisantes permettant l'évaluation du pouvoir cancérogène du TBP et on n'en a pas étudié les effets sur la fonction de reproduction.

L'aptitude du TBP à produire une neuropathie retardée n'a pas été suffisamment étudiée. Certes, les effets observés après administration orale d'une dose importante (0,42 ml/kg/jour pendant 14 jours) font songer à une neuropathie retardée, mais aucune dégénérescence n'a été relevée au niveau de axones et aucune conclusion définitive ne peut donc être tirée de ces études. A la même dose (0,42 ml/kg/jour pendant 14 jours) on a observé une réduction sensible de la vitesse de conduction au niveau du nerf caudal et une altération morphologique des fibres non myélinisées chez le rat. Ces résultats montrent que le TBP exerce des effets neurotoxiques sur les nerfs périphériques.

8. Effets sur l'homme

Lors d'une étude *in vitro*, on a relevé que le TBP avait un léger effet inhibiteur sur la cholinestérase plasmatique.

On n'a signalé aucun cas de neurotoxicité retardée comme cela est arrivé lors d'intoxications par le phosphate de tricrésyle.

EVALUATION DES RISQUES POUR LA SANTE HUMAINE ET DES EFFETS SUR L'ENVIRONNEMENT

1. Evaluation des risques pour la santé humaine

A part des maux de tête, des nausées et des symptômes d'irritation au niveau de la peau, des yeux et des muqueuses, on n'a pas signalé d'effets chez des personnes exposées de par leur profession. Aucun cas d'intoxication n'a été signalé dans la population générale.

Rien n'indique, compte tenu des résultats obtenus sur l'animal, que le TBP ait des effets neurotoxiques comparables à la neuropathie retardée que produisent les composés organophosphorés. Il est probable que la toxicité aiguë du TBP est faible pour l'homme.

Les résultats d'épreuves *in vitro* indiquent que le TBP n'est pas mutagène.

Le TBP est absorbé par voie cutanée, aussi faut-il éviter toute exposition de l'épiderme.

Des effets à long terme dus à une exposition professionnelle sont peu probables.

1.1 Niveaux d'exposition

Il y a probablement un risque d'exposition de la population générale au TBP par l'intermédiaire des divers compartiments de l'environnement et notamment par l'eau de consommation. Toutefois les concentrations de phosphate de tributyle mesurées dans de l'eau de boisson par l'Agence de Protection de l'Environnement des Etats-Unis se sont révélées extrêmement faibles et l'on a trouvé également des valeurs très basses au Canada et en Suisse. Des analyses effectuées aux Etats-Unis sur des tissus adipeux humains ont révélé la présence de traces de TBP dans un petit nombre d'échantillons. Cependant, les données sont insuffisantes pour qu'on puisse se faire une idée du degré d'exposition de la population générale au TBP.

Les personnes qui travaillent à l'entretien des aéronefs sont les plus exposées au TBP car elles sont amenées à manipuler des liquides hydrauliques qui en contiennent.

1.2 Effets toxiques

Le phosphate de tributyle peut pénétrer dans l'organisme par voie percutanée ou par ingestion. Toutefois, les données disponibles ne permettent pas de comparer utilement la pharmacocinétique de ces deux voies de pénétration.

A la lumière des données disponibles, il n'est pas possible d'évaluer le risque que constitue la TBP en tant qu'agent cancérogène, neurotoxique ou sensibilisant potentiel. Les observations qui font état d'une hyperplasie de l'épithélium vésical chez le rat, de signes de neurotoxicité (ataxie, incoordination, faiblesse, défaillance respiratoire) chez ce même animal et d'une sensibilisation chez les cobayes, ne paraissent pas suffisantes pour qu'on puisse procéder à une évaluation réelle du risque pour la santé humaine. On n'a pas observé de tumeur chez les rats. Chez les poulets, le TBP ne produit pas d'effets neurotoxiques retardés. En ce qui concerne la fonction de reproduction, les données disponibles ne sont pas suffisantes (qu'il s'agisse des gonades, de la fécondité, de la parturition ainsi que de la croissance et du développement des poussins).

2. Evaluation des effets sur l'environnement

Compte tenu de ses propriétés physicochimiques, le TBP présente une forte tendance à la bioaccumulation mais les mesures effectuées au laboratoire montrent qu'il n'en est rien dans la pratique. Les résidus présents dans la faune sauvage sont généralement faibles encore que la présence de résidus dosables chez certains oiseaux fasse songer à une possibilité de transfert par la chaîne alimentaire. Les données toxicologiques sont limitées mais indiquent une toxicité moyenne pour les organismes aquatiques. Toutes ces données tendent à confirmer l'opinion selon laquelle le TBP n'est guère dangereux pour les êtres vivants dans leur milieu naturel, du fait que les concentrations mesurées dans les eaux de surface sont généralement faibles.

2.1 Niveaux d'exposition

On trouve du TBP un peu partout dans les eaux super-
ficielles, les sédiments et les eaux souterraines mais en
principe sa concentration est faible. Dans l'eau, le TBP
subit une biodégradation aérobie appréciable mais celle-ci
est plutôt lente en-dessous de certaines concentrations.
Il est possible qu'il s'établisse un équilibre à faible
concentration dans le milieu naturel entre l'apport et
l'élimination du TBP. L'absence de données concernant la
vitesse d'hydrolyse du TBP ne permet pas d'évaluer de
façon fiable la persistance de ce produit dans
l'environnement. On ne peut donc pas déterminer le danger
potentiel que constitue cette substance. Il faudrait
avoir davantage de données sur la vitesse d'hydrolyse, ce
qui, compte tenu de ce que l'on sait de la biodégrabilité
du TBP, faciliterait l'évaluation de sa persistance et par
voie de conséquence, le risque qu'il constitue pour
l'environnement du fait de sa production, de son
utilisation et de son rejet.

2.2 Effets toxiques

Des épreuves statiques ont permis d'évaluer la
sensibilité des organismes aquatiques au TBP. Toutefois
ce produit étant biodégradable et relativement hydrophobe,
il serait bon d'effectuer des essais dans un courant
d'eau, ce qui permettrait d'obtenir des données plus
fiables en raison de la meilleure constance de l'exposition. Les données disponibles indiquent que le TBP est
modérément toxique pour les algues, les daphnies et la
truite arc-en-ciel. Il est dangereux pour les plantes
terrestres car il accroît la vitesse de dessication des
feuilles ce qui entraîne une défoliation excessive. On ne
dispose d'aucune donnée sur la fixation du phosphate de
tributyle ni sur sa translocation.

RECOMMANDATIONS

Il est nécessaire de poursuivre les travaux sur la sensibilisation cutanée par le phosphate de tri-*n*-butyle, sur sa tératogénicité et sur sa toxicité pour la fonction de reproduction, ainsi que sur sa pharmaco-cinétique selon différentes voies d'exposition.

Il est également nécessaire de poursuivre l'étude du pouvoir mutagène. Les épreuves *in vitro* initiales sur cultures de cellules mammaliennes devront si nécessaire être suivies d'épreuves *in vivo*. Selon les résultats de ces épreuves de mutagénicité, il pourra s'avérer nécessaire d'effectuer une étude de cancérogénicité.

RESUMEN

1. Identidad, propiedades físicas y químicas y métodos analíticos

El tri-*n*-butilfosfato (TBF) es un líquido no inflamable, no explosivo, incoloro e inodoro. Sin embargo, es térmicamente inestable y empieza a descomponerse a temperaturas inferiores a su punto de ebullición. Por analogía con las propiedades químicas conocidas del trimetilfosfato, se considera que el TBF se hidroliza rápidamente en soluciones ácidas, neutras o alcalinas. Se comporta como agente alquilizante débil. El coeficiente de reparto en etanol y agua (log P_{oa}) es de 3,99-4,01.

El método analítico más apropiado es la cromatografía gas-líquido con un detector sensible al nitrógeno-fósforo o un detector fotométrico de llama. El límite de detección en el agua es de unos 50 ng/litro. A menudo se han comunicado casos de contaminación de reactivos analíticos con TBF; por consiguiente, la obtención de datos fiables en el análisis de cantidades infinitesimales de TBF requiere un procedimiento cuidadoso.

2. Fuentes de exposición humana y ambiental

El TBF se obtiene mediante la reacción de *n*-butanol con oxicloruro de fósforo. Se utiliza como disolvente de ésteres de celulosa, lacas y gomas naturales, como plastificante primario en la fabricación de plásticos y de resinas vinílicas, como reactivo extractor de metales, como materia prima en la formulación de fluidos hidráulicos pirorresistentes para los aviones y como agente antiespumante. En los últimos años, ha aumentado de forma considerable la utilización del TBF como extractor en el proceso de disolución durante la reelaboración del combustible nuclear convencional.

La exposición de la población general por el uso normal puede considerarse mínima.

3. Transporte, distribución y transformación en el medio ambiente

Cuando se utiliza como reactivo extractor, disolvente o agente antiespumante se producen emisiones continuas de TBF al aire y al agua. La biodegradación del TBF es moderada o lenta, atendiendo al cociente entre su concentración y la biomasa activa. Consiste en una hidrólisis enzimática escalonada a ortofosfato y *n*-butanol, que experimenta una ulterior degradación. La concentración de TBF en el agua no disminuye con el empleo de las técnicas normales de tratamiento del agua de bebida.

Los factores de bioconcentración (FBC) medidos en dos especies de peces (*Fundulus* y *Carassius auratus*) oscilan entre 6 y 49. La semivida de depuración fue de 1,25 h.

4. Niveles medioambientales y exposición humana

Se ha detectado con frecuencia TBF en el aire, el agua, los sedimentos y los organismos acuáticos, pero los niveles en muestras medio ambientales son bajos. Se han encontrado concentraciones más altas de TBF en muestras de aire, agua y peces recogidas en las proximidades de instalaciones de fabricación de papel en el Japón: 13,4 ng/m^3 en el aire; 25 200 ng/litro en aguas fluviales; 111 ng/g en órganos de peces. Varios estudios de la dieta total realizados en el Reino Unido y los Estados Unidos indican un promedio diario de ingestión de TBF de unos 0,02-0,08 $\mu g/kg$ de peso corporal.

5. Efectos sobre los organismos vivos en el medio ambiente

Se ha calculado que las concentraciones inhibitorias (CE_0, CE_{50} y CE_{100}) de TBF para la multiplicación de algas unicelulares, protozoos y bacterias oscilan entre los 3,2 y los 100 mg/litro. La toxicidad aguda en los peces (CL_{50}) oscila entre 4,2 y 11,8 mg/litro. El TBF aumenta el ritmo de desecación en las hojas de las plantas, lo que origina una inhibición rápida y completa de la respiración foliar.

6. Cinética y metabolismo

En animales de experimentación, el TBF administrado por vía oral o por inyección intraperitoneal es rápidamente transformado en el hígado, y es de suponer que también en el riñón, para dar productos hidroxilados en forma de butilderivados. El TBF se excreta principalmente como dibutilhidrogenofosfato, butildihidrogenofosfato y butil bis-(3-hidroxibutil) fosfato. Los componentes alquílicos hidroxilados en forma de cadenas alquílicas se eliminan y excretan en parte como N-acetilalquilcisteína y en parte como anhídrido carbónico.

7. Efectos en los animales de experimentación y en sistemas de prueba *in vitro*

Se ha informado que, por vía oral, los valores de la DL_{50} del TFB en el ratón y ratas oscilan aproximadamente entre 1 y 3 g/kg, lo que indica una toxicidad aguda relativamente baja.

En estudios de toxicidad subcrónica con TBF se detectó una disminución en la ganancia de peso corporal y un aumento del peso del hígado, de los riñones y de los testículos. Los resultados de esos estudios indican que el riñón puede ser uno de los órganos destinatarios del TBF.

La irritación cutánea primaria que el TBF causa en los conejos albinos puede ser tan grave como la que produce la morfolina.

Se ha informado que, a dosis altas, el TBF puede ser ligeramente teratogénico. No se ha investigado suficientemente la mutagenicidad del TBF. Se han comunicado resultados negativos en pruebas con bacterias y en un ensayo de mutación letal recesiva con *Drosophila melanogaster*.

No hay datos suficientes para evaluar la actividad carcinogénica del TBF, y no se han investigado sus efectos sobre la reproducción.

No se ha investigado lo bastante la capacidad del TBF para producir neuropatía diferida. Los efectos observados después de la administración oral de una dosis alta (0,42 ml/kg diarios durante 14 días) indicaron una neuropatía diferida, pero no se detectó degeneración axonal y no se pudieron sacar conclusiones definitivas. Esta misma dosis alta (0,42 ml/kg diarios durante 14 días) causó una reducción importante en la velocidad de conducción del nervio caudal y una alteración morfológica de las fibras amielínicas de las ratas. Estos resultados indican que el TBF tiene un efecto neurotóxico en los nervios periféricos.

8. Efectos en la especie humana

Según un estudio *in vitro* el TBF tiene un efecto ligeramente inhibidor de la colinesterasa del plasma humano.

No se han notificado casos de neurotoxicidad diferida, como la observada en casos de intoxicación por tri-*o*-cresilfosfato.

EVALUACION DE LOS RIESGOS PARA LA SALUD HUMANA Y DE LOS EFECTOS EN EL MEDIO AMBIENTE

1. Evaluación de los riesgos para la salud humana

No se tienen noticias de que, en las personas profesionalmente expuestas, el TBF tenga otros efectos que dolor de cabeza, náuseas y síntomas de irritación de la piel, los ojos y las mucosas. No se han notificado casos de intoxicación entre la población general.

Los estudios con animales no indican que haya un efecto neurotóxico comparable a la neuropatía diferida que inducen los organofosfatos. La toxicidad sistémica en la especie humana después de una exposición intensa es probablemente baja.

De los resultados de las pruebas *in vitro* se deduce que el TBF no tiene efectos mutagénicos.

El TBF se absorbe a través de la piel, por lo que se debería limitar al máximo la exposición cutánea.

La probabilidad de que se observen efectos a largo plazo en las personas profesionalmente expuestas es pequeña.

1.1 Niveles de exposición

La población general puede estar expuesta al TBF en distintos medios ambientales, incluida el agua de bebidaC. Sin embargo, las concentraciones de TBF en el agua potable medidas por el Organismo de los Estados Unidos para la Protección del Medio Ambiente eran sumamente pequeñas; en el Japón, el Canadá y Suiza se han medido niveles igualmente bajos. En los EE.UU. se han llevado a cabo análisis de tejido adiposo humano que han revelado la existencia de indicios de TBF en un pequeño número de muestras. No hay datos suficientes para evaluar la importancia de la exposición de la población genereral al TBF.

Los trabajadores que se ocupan del mantenimiento de los aviones son, en potencia, el sector de la población más expuesto, a causa de la manipulación de fluidos hidráulicos que contienen TBF.

1.2 Efectos tóxicos

El tributilfosfato puede ingresar en el organismo por vía cutánea o por ingestión. Sin embargo, los datos disponibles no permiten establecer una comparación útil de la farmacocinética en ambas vías.

No se cuenta con información suficiente para evaluar el riesgo que representa el TBF como posible agente carcinogénico, neurotóxico o sensibilizante cutáneo. Las observaciones relativas a la inducción de hiperplasia del epitelio de la vejiga urinaria en la rata, a signos de neurotoxicidad (ataxia, falta de coordinación, debilidad y fallo respiratorio) en la misma especie y a sensibiliz-ación en el cobaya se consideran insuficientes para evaluar el peligro potencial del TBF para la salud humana. No se ha detectado en ratas la formación de tumores. El TBF no produce efectos neurotóxicos diferidos en la gallina. No se dispone de bastantes datos aacerca de los efectos del TBF en la reproducción (función de las gónadas, fertilidad, parto y crecimiento y desarrollo de la descendencia).

2. Evaluación de los efectos en el medio ambiente

Aunque en virtud de sus propiedades físico-químicas el TBF tiene un alto potencial de bioacumulación, las medidas efectuadas en los experimentos de laboratorio muestran que en la práctica no se bioacumula. Los residuos en las muestras de biota procedentes del medio ambiente son generalmente bajos, si bien los medidos en las aves ponen de manifiesto la posibilidad de una cierta transferencia en la cadena de alimentos. Los datos de toxicidad son limitados, pero indican que ésta es moderada para los organismos acuáticos. Esta información parece confirmar el critero de que el TBF entraña un riesgo mínimo para los seres vivos del medio ambiente, puesto que las concentraciones medidas en las aguas superficiales son generalmente bajas.

2.1 Niveles de exposición

Se ha encontrado TBF ampliamente distribuido en las aguas superficiales, los sedimentos y las aguas subterráneas, pero normalmente sólo en concentraciones bajas. La biodegradación del TBF en agua es considerable en condiciones aeróbicas, pero se verifica a escasa velocidad por debajo de determinadas concentraciones. Es posible que en la naturaleza se haya alcanzado un equilibrio para niveles bajos entre la liberación y la eliminación continuas. La falta de datos sobre la velocidad de hidrólisis del TBF impide valorar de manera fiable la persistencia del TBF en el medio ambiente. En consecuencia, no se puede evaluar el peligro potencial de la sustancia. Se necesitan más datos sobre la velocidad de hidrólisis del TBF que, junto con la información disponible sobre la biodegradabilidad, facilitarán la evaluación de su persistencia y, por consiguiente, el riesgo para el medio ambiente que representa su fabricación, uso y eliminación.

2.2 Efectos tóxicos

Se ha determinado la sensibilidad de los organismos acuáticos al TBF mediante pruebas estáticas. Sin embargo, sus características de biodegradabilidad y de relativa hidrofobicidad indican que los ensayos en corriente proporcionarían datos más fiables, debido a la exposición más constante. De la información disponible se deduce que el TBF tiene una toxicidad moderada para las algas, los dáfnidos y la trucha arco iris. El TBF causa lesiones en las plantas terrestres al aumentar la velocidad de desecación foliar, lo que conduce a una excesiva pérdida de hojas. No se dispone de datos acerca de su absorción y traslocación.

RECOMENDACIONES

Se necesitan más estudios sobre sensibilización cutánea, teratogenicidad y toxicidad en la reproducción, así como sobre la farmacocinética de las diferentes vías de exposición.

Hay que hacer más estudios para determinar la potencia mutagénica. Las pruebas iniciales *in vitro* en cultivos de células de mamíferos se deberían completar, en caso necesario, con pruebas *in vivo*. En función de los resultados de estas pruebas de mutagenicidad, puede ser necesario realizar un estudio de la carcinogenicidad.